# Consultation in Child and Adolescent Mental Health Services

Edited by

## Angela So

*Consultant Clinical Child Psychologist*
*Head of Child Psychology and Psychological Therapy Service*
*South Staffordshire Healthcare NHS Trust*

Foreword by

## Derek Steinberg

*Formerly Consultant Child and Adolescent Psychiatrist*
*Children's and Adolescents' Department*
*The Bethlem Royal and Maudsley Hospitals, London*

Radcliffe Publishing
Oxford • Seattle

**Radcliffe Publishing Ltd**
18 Marcham Road
Abingdon
Oxon OX14 1AA
United Kingdom

**www.radcliffe-oxford.com**
Electronic catalogue and worldwide online ordering facility.

---

© 2005 Angela Southall

British Library Cataloguing in Publication Data

A catalogue record for this book is available from the British Library.

ISBN 1 85775 800 5

Typeset by Anne Joshua & Associates, Oxford
Printed and bound by TJ International Ltd, Padstow, Cornwall

# Contents

# Foreword

Every so often a book comes along which makes a difference to thinking and practice, and I think this is one of them. Angela Southall and her collaborators have taken a subject which for many years has occupied the ambiguous position of being regarded as useful in child and adolescent mental health but also somewhat peripheral, and placed it centre stage. They have achieved this by highlighting in the clearest and most practical of ways aspects of work which are prominent in our daily practice and which consultative work is specifically designed to address.

In child mental health the traditional medical process of adding up the symptoms and signs and prescribing the treatment is the exception rather than the rule, the actual facts of daily practice being by no means so straightforward. For a start, many of the most frequently presenting problems, for example disturbances of mood, conduct and emerging personality, are not only grey areas, phenomenologically, but hotly disputed all the way from the family through the referring agents to potential helpers, and by experienced theoreticians and practitioners too. Exactly the same applies to the options for management. Further, where a problem or condition is eventually clarified, and the best way forward achieves consensus, it is usually precisely because a sufficiently broad view has been achieved, and because the clinical diagnosis, if there is one, has been widened out to demonstrate the influence of family, social, cultural, educational and biological factors, and who needs to do what about each – which can of course present new and sometimes difficult issues; but then no one said it should be easy.

Different practitioners deal with these real-life complexities in their own preferred ways, but it was the introduction of the notion of consultative work 30 or 40 years ago which usefully reframed the nature of our work, and showed that what seemed like a penumbra of cloudy issues getting in the way of clinical work was actually worthy of attention. It also helped clarify what was wrong and who and what could put things right, and as it happened was rather interesting as well.

Consultation – unfortunately a portmanteau term for all sorts of things, as Angela Southall discusses in her introduction – was designed and shaped as an adaptable tool for just this aspect of our work.

Probably most practitioners in child and adolescent mental health do some of their work broadly along consultative lines, just as most also undertake versions of counselling or psychotherapy shaped by personal experience, whatever study and training is behind it. But as work in any field evolves, a kind of natural selection operates in which the *ad hoc* in due course becomes the focus of more systematic attention, its principles clarified, practical experience reported, studies undertaken and the subject recognised and taught.

All this takes a long time. Family therapy, for example, has been developing within child and adolescent mental health for about 80 years, so that this thoroughly modern method is now not far from its Centenary. This kind of time scale is standard in the history of ideas, for example from quantum physics to computers, and as we know even Joseph Lister's ideas of 150 years ago about cleanliness in hospitals haven't yet quite caught on. Consultation as discussed in this book has been taking shape for some 30 or 40 years, so is relatively young, but I think it will take its place alongside other innovatory ideas and methods that have shaped our thinking. Angela Southall and her collaborators have produced a book which, with its clarity and its nice balance between principles and practicalities, is well-placed to give the subject the significant step forward it deserves in child and adolescent mental health and in wider aspects of healthcare practice too.

Derek Steinberg
Formerly Consultant Child and Adolescent Psychiatrist
Children's and Adolescents' Department
The Bethlem Royal and Maudsley Hospitals, London
*March 2005*

# About the editor

**Angela Southall** has been working with children, young people and families in an NHS setting since 1986. Since qualifying as a clinical psychologist she has sought to develop inter-disciplinary and interagency working and has been key in developing a number of community and interagency partnerships involving health, social care and education.

She leads a diverse multi-disciplinary Child Psychology and Psychological Therapy service in South Staffordshire. Her own clinical practice is in the fields of attachment and trauma and she is currently leading an Intensive Fostering project for young offenders, one of the first of its kind in the UK.

# List of contributors

**Rajeev Banhatti**, Consultant Child and Adolescent Psychiatrist, Child, Adolescent and Family Services, Northampton General Hospital NHS Trust

**Thelma Barlow**, SUSTAIN, Mill Bank Surgery, Mill Bank, Stafford

**Mandy Bryon**, Consultant Clinical Psychologist, Department of Psychological Medicine, Great Ormond Street Hospital, London

**Machita Denny**, Secretary, The Jigsaw Group, St George's Hospital, Stafford

**Kedar Nath Dwivedi**, Consultant Child and Adolescent Psychiatrist, Child, Adolescent and Family Services, Northampton General Hospital NHS Trust

**Louise Emanuel**, Child Psychotherapist, The Tavistock Clinic, London

**Kevin Epps**, Consultant Clinical and Forensic Psychologist; Honorary Lecturer, School of Psychology, University of Birmingham

**Michael Foulkes**, Systemic Psychotherapist and Consultant Family Therapist, Wolverhampton

**Fiona Gale**, CAMHS Regional Development Worker; CAMHS Programme Lead for NIMHE – East Midlands; National CAMHS Support Service, Leicester

**Evan George**, Solution-Focused Therapist

**Rita Harris**, Consultant Clinical Psychologist, The Tavistock Clinic, London

**Daniela Hearst**, Consultant Clinical Psychologist, Department of Psychological Medicine, Great Ormond Street Hospital, London

**Johanna Hilton**, Consultant Child and Forensic Psychologist, The Engage Service, Beaconside, Stafford

**Steve Jones**, Consultant Clinical Psychologist, Head of Child and Family Psychology and Psychotherapy, Sheffield Children's NHS Trust

**Dave Poole**, Trainee Social Worker, Cannock Social Services, Staffordshire

**Emma Probert**, Young People's Focus Group, Cannock Chase CAMHS, Cannock, Staffordshire

**Scott Sinclair**, Clinical Psychologist, South Staffordshire Healthcare NHS Trust; Honorary Research Fellow, University of Birmingham

**Angela Southall**, Consultant Clinical Child Psychologist; Head of Child Psychology and Psychological Therapy Service, South Staffordshire Healthcare NHS Trust

**Caitlyn Staples**, Young People's Focus Group, Cannock Chase CAMHS, Cannock, Staffordshire

**Kate Stokes**, SUSTAIN, Mill Bank Surgery, Mill Bank, Stafford

**Donna Wedgbury**, Associate Director, South Staffordshire Healthcare NHS Trust, St George's Hospital, Stafford

In memory of Scott Sinclair 1971–2003.

# Introduction

## What is mental health?

Often, when children's mental health needs are discussed, what follows tends to be framed around mental ill health, rather than well-being. What do we mean by mental health? A recent definition by the Mental Health Foundation (Kay 1999) suggests that children who have good mental health show this in their capacity to do a number of things, namely:

- to develop psychologically, emotionally, intellectually and spiritually
- to initiate, develop and sustain mutually satisfying personal relationships
- to use and enjoy solitude
- to become aware of others and empathise with them
- to play and learn
- to develop a sense of right and wrong
- to resolve (face) problems and setbacks and learn from them.

Children's mental health services are set up to facilitate all elements pertaining to emotional well-being and have a very significant preventative role. They are often unable to fulfil this role as demands for services have, year on year, outstripped resources, resulting in many services finding themselves in a position of feeling they can do little more than 'fire-fighting'. As part of an examination of children's health services across the nation, the Department of Health (DoH) has refocused concern on the mental health and psychological well-being of children and young people through the National Service Framework (NSF) for Children (DoH 2003). This document has a focus on achieving common standards across the country and developing services through improvement, investment, expansion and reform over a ten-year period. It states the aims of child and adolescent mental health services as being:

> to meet the needs and views of children and young people with mental health problems, together with those of their families and carers, in order to improve their life chances . . .

> [Services should] respect difference and diversity, take into account the best available evidence for effectiveness, and [be] delivered within a reasonable timeframe and in an appropriate setting by a competent, skilled and supported multidisciplinary workforce.

The NSF for Children tells us there are 12 million children in England, 400 000 of whom are officially classified as 'children in need'. Approximately 1 million children have mental health problems (DoH 2003). A great many children, therefore, do not enjoy good mental health. Although there is some variation in the literature, the general consensus seems to be that up to 25% of children experience a mental health problem (Kramer and Garralda 2000), with incidences being higher in some groups than others, such as looked-after children or

1

children with chronic illnesses. Social status continues to be a major indicator of mental health status (Meltzer *et al.* 2000).

## The context of child and adolescent mental health services

Child and adolescent mental health services – commonly abbreviated to the acronym CAMHS – is a term used to describe the spectrum of services provided around children's mental health. Services range from those provided by voluntary agencies and non-specialist health, education and social care practitioners to mental health professionals, dedicated mental health teams and highly specialist services, such as therapeutic units. Unfortunately, as is common in health, there is room for confusion, as the term CAMHS is also used simultaneously to describe the community CAMHS teams, working mainly in and around the tier 2 level. Across the country, these teams often refer to themselves simply as 'CAMHS teams'. In order to differentiate such teams from the wide range of CAMH services, where appropriate this text will refer to these multidisciplinary health teams as 'community CAMHS teams'.

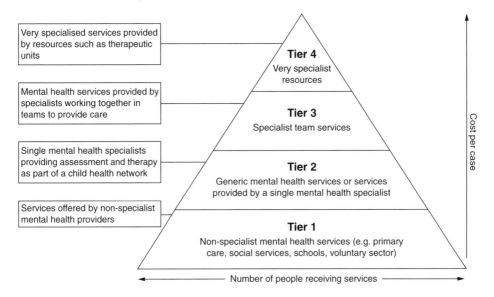

Figure A Child and adolescent mental health services tiered structure.

## Recent developments in CAMHS

In recent years there has been increasing diversification of therapeutic approaches offered in the specialist child and adolescent mental health services (CAMHS), through multidisciplinary community CAMHS teams, specialist networks and single-discipline providers. Organised in an increasing number of ways, community CAMHS teams are usually able to offer a 'menu' of therapies from which different elements may be selected or combined, according to need.

These include psychiatric and other medical approaches, family and systemic therapies, creative therapies, psychotherapy and counselling, and a range of psychological therapies, such as cognitive behaviour therapy. The term 'direct work' is sometimes used to describe these therapeutic methods of working, as the practitioner works directly with the client and significant others, such as his or her carers.

Direct (assessment and therapeutic) work is only part of a much wider brief to provide specialist mental health services to children, young people and their families. This wider brief includes development, liaison and support services, teaching, training and consultation. As demands for services have grown, so also have the indirect methods, with some interesting and exciting results. There has been a shift away from merely increasing the number of specialist practitioners in order to try to meet ever-growing needs. Instead, indirect methods have begun to be acknowledged, not just as an add-on but as a credible and integral part of services. A number of such initiatives focus on community partnerships, enhancing the skills of non-specialists through training and consultation. Their success has supported a growing view among specialist practitioners that in order to begin to make any real impact we need to radically rethink the way we work.

Consultation is just one of a number of ways that specialist CAMHS practitioners can help each other, as well as their colleagues in the non-specialist field. It offers significant opportunities to 'change the map' of service provision and delivery. Although consultation may be used very successfully in a number of settings and situations, this book will focus on its applications to child and adolescent mental health work.

## What is consultation?

It is important to think about what is meant by this umbrella term 'consultation' as it is a word with numerous definitions. The title of 'consultant' has many meanings in western culture and is simultaneously used to describe a number of different things. A medical consultant, for example, though having that particular title, rarely, if ever, functions as a consultant, in the sense used in this book. Likewise, the term 'consultation' may be used to describe a number of different personal transactions, from a general practitioner (GP) appointment to a financial or therapeutic one. Traditionally, the term implies some sort of advice- or help-giving relationship between consultee (the person seeking advice) and consultant (the person giving it).

The definition adopted by this book is that consultation is an activity in which one practitioner helps another through a process of joint enquiry and exploration. The work discussed remains the responsibility of the consultee, who retains control of its direction, decision making and methodologies. If there is a problem to be solved, it is the consultee and not the consultant who has the responsibility of solving it: the focus of the consultation is the process of the work itself, not the problem. The consultation therefore emphasises mutuality, requiring the consultant to adopt a collaborative position with the consultee, rather than an expert one.

This is not easy, for either party. Professional culture expectations tend to organise themselves around ideas of 'expertness'. This is especially pronounced in the field of health. It can be hard for those taking on the role of consultant to adopt a new role that is in many ways quite alien to their training and professional ethos. Similarly, consultees entering into the consultation relationship may find it hard to resist their strong desire to be told what to do. For both individuals, the compulsion to resume old roles can be strong and anxiety levels high. In short, it is not an easy relationship to enter into. As Steinberg (1989) writes:

> 'To consult' is the word for what both consultant and consultee do, and both require skill to do it.

## Supervision

Although the varied accounts of consultation in diverse settings provided by each of the contributors to this text distinguish it from the process of supervision, it needs to be emphasised that supervision and consultation are distinct processes (*see* Table 1). Whereas consultation is based on equality and mutual exploration, the supervisory relationship is characterised essentially by differences in seniority, with the supervisor holding a more senior and responsible position. Usually, when supervision is set up within an organisation or agency context, the more senior professional will have (ultimate) responsibility for the work.

The supervisory relationship is very clearly centred around the supervisor helping the supervisee with his or her work whilst also maintaining an overview of quality standards, clinical competence and case management. In effect, this is really supervision of the *person* through the work they present. The critical issue is the balance of power and who has the responsibility. If this is in any doubt, it is easily answered by asking who has to address the complaint when things go wrong.

The exception to this is peer supervision, where two or more practitioners meet to discuss the details of their practice. Here the focus is on helping each other. Those involved in peer supervision are typically of the same professional background or discipline. In the field of specialist mental health, peer supervision is usually an adjunct to the sort of clinical supervision described above.

**Table 1** Therapy, supervision and consultation matrix

| *Relationship* | *Power/responsibility* | *Focus* |
| --- | --- | --- |
| Therapy | Therapist | Client |
| Supervision | Supervisor | Supervisee |
| Consultation | Consultee | Practice/organisation |

# The advantages of consultation

Consultation benefits services in a number of ways, some of which are listed below:

- Consultation is a mutual learning process, leading to intra and interprofessional development, including service development.
- The unique perspective (i.e. that of the consultee) is inherently validating of the consultee's skills.
- Consultation enhances skills across groups of professionals, rather than in one individual. The focus on the skills and understanding of the consultee facilitates the identification of training and other needs. Either serially or in groups, the process enables a number of professionals to benefit in this way.
- Consultation can prevent the ongoing referral (or re-referral) of a proportion of children, young people and families (sometimes a sizeable one) by enabling them to stay with their original 'front-line' practitioner.
- At the same time, it can also speed the process of accessing more specialist help, when necessary, by helping to clarify and make specific the reasons for doing so.
- Consultation is an activity that helps build relationships between individuals, areas of service and agencies. It can be seen therefore as one of the essential facilitators of a 'working together' philosophy.
- Finally, consultation provides an opportunity to take advantage of the increased diversification of CAMHS *outside* of specialist teams and maximise opportunities for making a difference.

# The need for new considerations

Consultation is not a new idea and has been around in one way or another for a number of years, during which time it has evolved into a very distinct practice. It is notable, however, that professional training for mental health practitioners has not kept pace with this very important development. Training courses fail to include consultation, both at the conceptual and practice levels. Similarly, the literature does not reflect the development or ascendancy of consultation. Caplan (1970) continues to be the most cited, despite its vintage. More recent texts (e.g. Fritz *et al.* 1993) promote a view of the consultant as an expert and focus on consultation as advice giving rather than as a facilitative, enabling relationship. Others, although emphasising the uniqueness and the egalitarian nature of the consultation relationship, nevertheless covertly maintain this position (e.g. Wynne *et al.* 1986). With the exception of Steinberg (1989), the literature reveals a striking adherence to Caplan's (1970) view of the consultant 'working through' the consultee, thereby betraying a view that it is really the consultant – and not the consultee – that does the work.

   Given the current impetus to work more effectively and efficiently, a fresh look at consultation is timely.

   This book considers consultation in different settings which themselves highlight specific issues and illustrate particular aspects of the work. In this way, theory and practice are interwoven to inform each other through the chapters. Steve Jones and Fiona Gale describe two different ways of delivering primary care consultation. This is followed by Louise Emanuel's account of psychodynamic consultation in two very different educational settings and Evan George's description of solution-focused consultation with the staff of a 'failing' school. There follows a social services focus, with a chapter describing consultation at the social services area office, which includes a detailed case study of an 18-month ongoing piece of consultation work. Michael Foulkes then challenges the reader to integrate political and theoretical issues in the story of his consultation to the mother of two sexually abused children. Rajeev Banhatti and Kedar Dwivedi go on to describe psychiatric consultation through the community CAMHS team, considering a range of consultation settings that are encountered. There follows a chapter by Mandy Bryon and Daniela Hearst illustrating paediatric psychology consultation. The specialist forensic field is represented by two chapters: the first, by Scott Sinclair and Kevin Epps, describes their work in the community with youth offending teams; the second chapter, by Johanna Hilton, gives an account of her experiences as a consultant to a local authority children's secure home. Rita Harris then shares her experiences of teaching consultation skills, focusing on managers as consultants. We then hear from service user-consultants themselves about their experiences. The final chapter will synthesise ideas in order to suggest a new and more comprehensive model of consultation that enables future directions for consultation in children's services to emerge.

This is not a definitive list of potential consultation 'areas', which are limited only by the imagination and creativity of all of us who practise. Neither is it a 'how to' book. Rather, it aims to cover the main areas of CAMHS consultation across the 'tiers' and promote enthusiasm in practitioner and manager alike. If you are already consulting with other professionals as part of your practice, I hope you find this book interesting and inspiring to do more. If you are not, I hope you find the fascinating accounts of other people's work in this book encourage you to have a go. Good luck.

Angela Southall
*March 2005*

# References

Caplan G (1970) *The Theory and Practice of Mental Health Consultation*. Tavistock Publications, London.

Fritz GK, Mattison RE, Nurcombe B *et al.* (1993) *Child and Adolescent Mental Health Consultation in Hospitals, Schools and Courts*. American Psychiatric Press, Washington, DC.

Department of Health (2003) *Getting the Right Start: the National Service Framework (NSF) for Children, Young People and Maternity – emerging findings*. HMSO, London.

Kay H (1999) *Bright Futures: promoting children and young people's mental health*. The Mental Health Foundation, London.

Kramer T and Garralda EM (2000) Child and adolescent mental health problems in primary care. *Advances in Psychiatric Treatment*. **6**: 287–94.

Meltzer, Gatward, Goodman *et al.* (2000) *Mental Health of Children and Adolescents in Great Britain*. HMSO, London.

Steinberg D (1989) *Inter-professional Consultation*. Blackwell Scientific Publications, Oxford.

Wynne LC, McDaniel SH and Weber TT (eds) (1986) *Systems Consultation: a new perspective for family therapy*. Guilford Press, New York.

# Chapter 1

# Good practice: consultation to a primary care team

*Steve Jones*

## Introduction

Consultation has sometimes been described in terms that betray a view of the process of consultation as the expert working through the consultee (e.g. Caplan 1970), rather than facilitating or enabling within the consultee's frame of reference and context. This chapter describes a consultation experience with a multidisciplinary primary care team of general practitioners (GPs), health visitors, a community psychiatric nurse and other staff who were attached to the practice. This is an attempt to reflect the experiences of both the consultant and the primary care team and to illustrate the context and practice benefits.

## Consultation from a general practice perspective

This account is of a regular consultation meeting that evolved with one general practice team over approximately ten years. A 'consultation workshop' developed with the multidisciplinary primary care team, which itself also changed and evolved over time, with members leaving and joining, visitors coming and going, whilst very substantial changes impacted on the practice itself and upon its members' professional lives. During this time, all but one of the practice GP principals changed, team members retired or took sabbaticals, and major changes affected the practice itself: physical changes took place as the building was redesigned and developed; strategic and organisational changes in the National Health Service (NHS) were reflected in services offered. The practice was a belated convert to 'GP fund-holding' which gave the staff much more local control over their patients' healthcare provision. This was subsequently extended as they became a personal medical services (PMS) pilot. Both these latter changes not only gave the practice opportunities to innovate in healthcare with more control over the services it provided, but also meant that it had an economic interest in the outcomes of the consultation workshop as well as a health interest.

The consultation workshop was established from a primary care perspective and the content or focus of sessions was very much defined by the primary care team itself. It was not organised around specific categories or groups of individuals such as 'the under-fives'; neither did it define itself in terms of specialist secondary healthcare notions of a separating out into distinct category topics such as child and adolescent mental health. Consultation cases could be drawn from the full age range and many were singularly not defined by a 'mental health' label – the primary concern being on different occasions the patient's physical health, their pattern of attendance or use of practice and NHS healthcare resources. Nonetheless, the consultant's expertise in human behaviour and relationships was an important resource and there was a natural bias in the content of the consultation towards the specialist interest of the consultant which was child and family mental health.

## A consultation workshop?

Consultations took place during a regular meeting between an experienced clinical child psychologist who was also a systemic family therapist and members of the general practice primary care team. In the initial few meetings only doctors attended but, almost immediately, the practice-attached health visitors and community psychiatric nurse joined too. Over time, all of the practice doctors joined the workshop, together with trainees, other primary care staff such as the school nurse, practice nurses and, occasionally, local voluntary organisations.

The workshop took place monthly as a lunch-time meeting lasting approximately one and a half hours over a sandwich lunch which was always provided. Initially, there was a commitment to discussing three cases per workshop but, over time, the focus was more likely to be a lengthy conversation over a single case, occasionally an entire extended family or a theme, such as substance misuse. Individual practitioners selected cases for the consultation. Usually, but not invariably, the selection was agreed by the team before the meeting. The concerns addressed in the consultation workshop included:

- behavioural and emotional problems affecting children or adults
- family difficulties
- treatment management problems (e.g. non-adherence to treatment, inappropriate secondary referrals)
- problems in a patient's use of the practice itself (e.g. excessive or inappropriate out-of-hours calls)
- problems regarding a patient's relationship with the practice team
- any 'stuck' or 'heart-sink' case.

In describing the consultation workshop, we debated how to label it. The process was felt to share many of the characteristics of supervision, in that it was a facilitated, scheduled case discussion forum with a specific, small group of professionals. However, there were some important differences. For example, the facilitator-consultant explicitly lacked much of the knowledge and skills required and used by team members and responsibility for any case-work remained very clearly with the individual practitioner or practice team, with cases being rarely revisited. Initially, implicit expectations were perhaps more akin to supervision wherein there might be an expectation that practice would be validated by the 'expert supervisor'. Our explicit contract refocused this very rapidly into a much more complementary consultation process which later evolved, as discussed below, into a form of co-consultation.

---

Case study 1.1

One of the general practitioners was concerned about two children in the same family who were not complying with asthma therapy. In consequence their condition was unstable with repeated visits to the surgery and what was considered to be an excessive number of out-of-hours call-outs. The consultation workshop revealed, *inter alia*, that one of the parents, who usually saw a different GP for her own health concerns, had Crohn's disease and had become 'cushingoid' due to steroid therapy. The team hypothesised that, in consequence, the children were not being supported to comply effectively with their own steroid treatment. The outcome of the consultation was a revised multidisciplinary treatment approach that included 'educational' counselling for the parents.

---

## Before beginning

The consultation workshop was initiated following contributions made to general practitioner training by the consultant and in the context of the primary care team's existing commitment to working and learning together – particularly about their own consulting relationships with their patients. The GP vocational training scheme co-ordinator was based in the practice and championed the consultation workshop. The practice team already had regular practice meetings and they had also made a previous, brief and challenging attempt at group consultation. Of the latter, team members said they had learnt from the process but it was highly stressful, often leaving them anxious and literally in a sweat at the prospect of presenting their case or being 'psychoanalysed' themselves. The type of experiences alluded to are reminiscent of an approach dubbed 'therapeutic' supervision by Rosenblatt and Mayer (1975). This has been reported by supervisees as their least popular approach. It seemed important to distinguish the new venture from the last with more emphasis on safety, inclusiveness and facilitation.

## Beginning consultation: contracting

An initial contract was agreed for just three consultation sessions, specifying that up to three cases would be consulted to per session, determined wholly by the consultees according to what concerned them. It was agreed that the sessions needed to be made 'safe', giving a clear brief that this would be a relaxed, 'atheoretical' workshop focused on facilitating the team members' existing way of working and that consultees would not themselves be the subject of personal or therapeutic interpretations. As a local secondary healthcare professional, it was also agreed that the workshop would not be a forum for expediting referrals and nor would the consultant offer 'expert' opinion or teaching in his area of clinical expertise.

The initial contract was with three general practitioners but the agreement explicitly invited all others in the practice to join. Having reviewed the sessions, the contract was extended for a further six months and then extended indefinitely, although periodic reviews continued to be held.

---

**Case study 1.2**

One health visitor was concerned about a family where Laurie, aged nine, had Duchenne muscular dystrophy. Anne, Laurie's mother, was extremely anxious. The team, with the GP who was principally involved, focused on the family secrets that had built up around the diagnosis, Anne's own understanding of the disease, and Laurie's needs and risks. The outcome of the consultation was agreement to undertake a team approach whereby the health visitor and one of the GPs planned how they might help to break the news and support the family subsequently.

---

## The consultation process

Consultation to a mixed discipline group is less able to rely on assumptions about shared values, understanding about good practice, ethical codes and group manners (Proctor and Inskipp 2001). In this case the group was also a work team with its own history, established professional codes of expectation and behaviour as well as personal interactions within and outside of the workplace.

The process of consulting to, or supervising, a natural work team, rather than a group drawn together for this purpose, acknowledges, in particular, the team members' considerable knowledge about their setting, their different skills and also the different roles of team members and their relationships with each other outside of the consultation workshop. In contrast to uniprofessional group supervision, the different roles, expertise and informal hierarchy made an important contribution to the working of the consultation workshop.

What emerged as a unique aspect of consulting to a multidisciplinary primary care team was that, although a particular case would be presented by an individual practitioner, other members of the team were likely to have a current, intercurrent or previous involvement with the patient. Often team members would have information about prior episodes sometimes years before or about key members of the extended family or community which may extend back two or more generations. The outcome of any particular consultation might therefore include not only other team members' information but also their professional knowledge and skills, potentially leading to a significantly revised cast of professionals leading the healthcare intervention.

## Team foundations and consultation champion

This primary care team possessed some crucial characteristics to support and make use of the consultation workshop: the general practitioners and other practice team members had experience of meeting as a team, there was already some history of discussing clinical topics, they had a commitment to learning together and to improving their practice. This context provided the foundations for a good working group for the consultation workshop. Proctor and Inskipp (2001) characterised a good working group as having the following qualities:

• feeling safe enough with each other and with the consultant to trust the group with honest disclosure of their work

- clarity about the task
- knowing each other well enough as individuals
- accepting and respecting difference
- sharing sufficient values, beliefs and assumptions about human beings and professional helping
- 'good group manners'.

In addition to responding to the team's relationships and the changes in them, one of the key informal roles in the consultation workshop was that of 'consultation champion'. Although team members have been variously enthusiastic or enthused, experience suggests that a team consultation relies on its being championed by one of the senior team members who ensures that the space is protected and supported organisationally. It is crucial to understanding the success of *this* consultation workshop that the workshop had an internal team champion at the outset and was then able to build on, develop and maintain the characteristics of a good working group despite many changes and upheavals.

Making consultation safe was a key task although it is also important to reiterate that this team was brave enough and comfortable enough with each other to begin at all. The consultant acted to avoid blaming, to create boundaries around the subject matter, to include all members of the team and created an opportunity to share feelings about difficult, complex and 'stuck' cases. Validating both feelings and actions was an important outcome for team members, whilst from time to time the team champion also needed support in being 'one of the team' whilst continuing to validate their role as 'consultation champion'.

---

**Case study 1.3**

Billy, an eight-year-old 'livewire' who was always up to mischief, had already been suspended from school when he died, having fallen off a wall whilst in the care of his stepfather, David. Three months later the family health visitor was concerned for each of the family members: David blamed himself but couldn't talk about what had happened; Billy's mum also blamed herself and couldn't stop talking about it outside the family, whilst his sister, Natasha, looked sad and lost. The health visitor with the team reviewed the family's circumstances, how they had responded to and communicated about the death and its aftermath. A hypothesis was developed that family members had become completely isolated as individuals, that no one in the family knew how to speak to each other anymore and the mourning process had become 'stuck'. After some planning and rehearsal, the very experienced health visitor agreed that she and the family had the strengths to move on and that she would convene a meeting with the family to help them start to communicate once more about their loss and its meaning.

---

## Facilitating the consultation workshop

The consultant's key contribution was to provide a consistent context with a clear focus, within which all team members were encouraged to contribute. It was also important to be clear about the limits to the consultant's expertise – that this 'expert' was no such thing in relation to many of the team's tasks (for example, health visiting or medical practice) or the local community context – and to maintain the 'consultative' stance. An important role was to encourage reflexivity and contributions from within the team, enlisting colleagues in contributing to the thinking around the issues. Conversely, because the local community child and adolescent mental health services (CAMHS) included this practice, it was also important to respond to invitations to enlist the consultant as an expert to whom a referral might be made.

Supported by the internal champions and the commitment of the team itself, the tasks of the consultant in the consultation workshop are shown in Box 1.1.

For a multidisciplinary primary care team some aspects acquired more prominence, namely, structuring thinking in an integrated way, drawing in other practitioners' knowledge and experience, and connecting client and family history. The latter was often important for general practitioners, who experienced only very brief disjointed appointments, sometimes scattered across different practitioners. The effect of connecting these observations – expounding the individual patient's story, the family and community context and, indeed, the team context – was often to 'reframe' the initial presenting problem, creating a new, richer story or 'narrative' for the individual practitioner and the team (Launer 2002).

The style of consultation that evolved included processes of:

- exploration and collaboration – clarifying with contributions from the team
- support – being non-judgemental and encouraging the team to contribute supportively
- assessment – reviewing in the team that appropriate primary care assessments and checks had been completed
- intervention – planning a team approach (which, as the workshop evolved, might include the consultant's skills too but as one member of the team)
- validating – confirming that all reasonable steps had been taken and that the lead practitioner's feelings were shared and understood
- no personal therapy or personal interpretations

---

**Box 1.1 Consultation workshop: tasks of the consultant**

- Chairing the conversation
- Clarifying the reason and timing for concern
- Structuring the thinking of participants around the case
- Facilitating a new and holistic consideration of complex and stuck cases
- Ensuring that all team members were able to contribute
- Making space to reflect, to feel and to make connections
- Leading the conversation in directions that had not been considered
- Drawing out the reflexive (circular) nature of some relationships
- Facilitating the construction of a new 'narrative' or revised formulation for the case
- Leading towards concluding action points or confirming and validating actions already undertaken

- no teaching
- not treating the consultant as a fount of expert knowledge
- not treating the workshop as a referral meeting (although referral could be one outcome).

A key aspect of consultation or supervision is the extent to which the relationships between and amongst consultant and consultees can sustain and respond to challenges to the consultee's existing thoughts, feelings or frame of reference. Implicit in the early contract was an expectation that the challenge would be respectful and supportive. Over time, the strength of challenge offered or facilitated in this team consultation evolved and related to the degree of comfort with the consultant, the current 'health' of the team and the changes going on within it.

---

**Case study 1.4**

The practice realised that it was responding to a rapidly increasing influx of patients from another part of the country who were registered drug addicts. The patients appeared to form an extended community, living in relatively isolated, rented cottages. Consultation clarified that the practice team had not encountered this as a significant health concern before and were concerned about their capacity and skills to respond to this new group of patients who had swiftly reached 16 in number. Further anxieties focused on child protection concerns for some families and an increased risk of local youngsters being inducted into substance misuse.

   The kernel of an action plan was developed for the practice as a whole and which included other agencies. This included evidence-based research and contacting for advice a local specialist GP and the specialist substance misuse service. The primary care trust was approached to ensure that health records were swiftly obtained and a policy devised to address, *inter alia*, these patients' health consulting (named doctors only), prescribing, reception support and waiting room behaviour. Multi-agency liaison included social services regarding child protection, benefits and housing issues as well as youth services.

   As a consequence of the consultation opportunity, the practice team was able to orchestrate a swift, holistic response to this unfamiliar challenge which took account of their own learning needs as well as, for example, the health, social care, housing and community issues. The consultation workshop in this case was simply the first of a series of practice meetings and multi-agency and community liaison.

---

## Evaluating the primary care team consultation workshop: does it help?

Initial and periodic team reviews of the consultation workshop were undertaken and individual feedback invited, including from 'leavers', although the workshop was not externally evaluated. The workshop was subject to regular joint review by a practice that was astute in managing its resources, including this monthly meeting which was relatively expensive of their time. At one level the continuation of the consultation workshop over many years suggests of itself that both the practice team and consultant gained from the relationship. Unsurprisingly, in view of that history, participants commented that the workshop was not only helpful but enjoyable and a safe place to verbalise anxieties.

Collective evaluation of the consultation workshop asserted that it contributed to improving the health of individual patients and the health of their families. The team's experience was that it helped to broaden and structure their approach, integrating physical, psychological and social aspects of healthcare for the more complex cases.

The team consultation approach offered an overview in respect of patients or circumstances where services appeared ineffective, inappropriate or excessive. The consultation workshop was thought by the team to be effective in helping to restructure formulations and intervention packages both from individual practitioners and from the team as a whole. As well as improving patient care, some unnecessary referrals and investigations were also averted. Evaluation of some individual cases suggested that the approach sometimes saved substantial resources, either by improving effectiveness, reducing inappropriate use of team resources or by obviating expensive, sometimes demonstrably ineffective, secondary care referrals.

Participant reports for a mid-point evaluation after four years of the workshop suggested that the approach had had an impact on the relationship with patients, supporting practitioners with chronic or 'heart-sink' patients and halting the potential breakdown in doctor–patient relationships. The workshop was seen to facilitate a more objective view of the practitioner–patient relationship or helped actively to punctuate that relationship in a different way. Participants thought this could interrupt a spiral of decline which often leads to disillusionment or even, *in extremis*, to patients being asked to leave the practice list. The latter eventuality was never reached in the ten years of the workshop but it was noteworthy that the topic was raised or alluded to in some of the cases brought for consultation and prior to the consultation workshop commencing patients had been 'de-listed'.

A very important outcome in some consultations was simply the opportunity to verbalise anxieties, particularly about chronic or stuck cases, in a non-threatening environment. This was often supported by the team's validation that the consultee was doing all that could reasonably be done in the circumstances of the case and that their feelings were shared.

This practice had a strong learning ethos and a commitment to new ways of working across disciplines which the workshop further supported, facilitating a more reflexive practice and challenging preconceived ideas and assumptions: team members reported that they learned much about each other's roles and contributions and much from each other. Individual practitioners were supported in changing their personal stance, for example in withdrawing from the temptation to adopt the position of 'rescuer'. Some incidental learning also took place and, although this was not a systemic practice teaching workshop, many of the practice now make some use of, for example, the genogram as a basic tool.

All participants in the consultation workshop commented on its positive impact on the practice team itself. They also felt that the workshop had a team-building function, extending their understanding of each other's roles and skills and improving morale. The workshop also reduced feelings of isolation, pooling the knowledge of team members and facilitating more cohesive intervention.

The consultation workshop also illustrated to the consultant, ensconced in the rarified world of specialist mental healthcare, the complexity and chronicity of some of the work undertaken within primary care which does not always sit easily within the specialist divisions of secondary healthcare.

---

**Case study 1.5**

One of the general practitioners was concerned about Martina, whose husband had died following an asthma attack seven years previously. Over the past 12 months she had been making increasingly frequent, approximately fortnightly, unplanned visits to the surgery, sometimes bringing her 15-year-old son, Matthew. Matthew had 'gone off the rails' since his father's death, having being suspended from school, and was getting into trouble with the police. Most of Matthew's consultations related to his mother's difficulty in coping with him or police involvement. The family was relatively affluent but socially isolated. Martina herself tended to be anxious and she was alternately overprotective of, or over-reliant on, her two teenage children.

The workshop revealed that 17-year-old Tanya consulted different partners in the practice but, like her mother, also with increasing frequency in connection with a range of vague complaints. Tanya was said to be a quiet young woman but her mother was concerned that she had taken up with an 'unsuitable' older man.

Martina herself had had a very serious infection since her husband's death from which she had fully recovered, but at the time it had resulted in her near death and admission to an intensive treatment unit. Since her husband's death she had also experienced several episodes of severe depression which had responded to antidepressant medication but relapsed when the medication was stopped.

Although some time had elapsed since the family's bereavement, the workshop hypothesised that some of the difficulties lay in the unresolved bereavement. Martina's GP had become used to a sequence of brief and unsatisfactory, superficially unconnected, consultations. He determined to punctuate this with a planned, longer meeting where he would try to rebuild a deeper rapport with Martina and take stock with her of her loss and the ensuing years. He would also enter the meeting supported by the community psychiatric nurse's offer to convene a family meeting to help him address this if appropriate.

---

## Beginning: establishing the consultation workshop

The initial phase of the consultation workshop was setting up and 'joining' an initial explorative exercise with just three practice members, which swiftly became a multidisciplinary conversation including at different times most practitioner staff and trainees. At the outset it had been agreed that the three practitioners present would proceed in any event in order to fulfil their own aims but that the invitation to other practice staff to participate would be reiterated. Consequently, within two to six meetings the core membership of six practitioners – notwithstanding subsequent staff changes – was established. It was agreed after the second planned review at nine months that the exercise seemed worthwhile and would be continued with periodic reviews.

The role of internal champion was crucial in the workshop's success – as it often is in establishing similar groups within work teams. From the outset a senior GP championed the consultation workshop and was always supported by at least one other member of the team in this informal role. Success was evident not only in the 'administrative support' provided but also in organising attendance, planning cases for discussion prior to the meeting and in consistent attendance and contributions. The internal organisational support provided by the practice was also vital – reliably offering a consistent, comfortable time and space to meet sustained by a sandwich lunch.

The joining phase was characterised by a conscious respect on the consultant's part for the different and overlapping expertise of the participants coupled with a concern to achieve good 'group manners'. At this stage the focus was on the individual practitioner presenting the case, ensuring that their needs were met and that the workshop also achieved the target of three cases for consultation at each session.

## Learning: developing a cyclical model of consultation

The second phase of the workshop involved a stable multidisciplinary staff group and continued for some two years (until several significant practice staff retired or left). This second phase was characterised by attempts to include all participants in the workshop, not merely in presenting cases for consultation but also in drawing on the knowledge they held about the case history and context, often over many years. This also appeared to be a time when participants were themselves learning more about each other's professional roles and skills as some had not worked as such a close primary care team before. During both these phases the consultant continued to define a role as 'consultant' rather than 'expert supervisor' or as someone through whom referrals might be expedited. This is not to say that expedition of referrals might not be one of the roles or functions of others who consult to primary care (or 'tier 1') professionals, such as primary mental health workers in child and mental health services (*see* Chapter 2).

During the second phase an emphasis developed towards creating a different understanding or 'narrative' around just one or two cases rather than seeking new solutions for three. This, the creation of a richer, more joined-up account, initially seemed a profligate luxury imported from the 'indulgence' of psychological therapy, but it gave GPs especially the opportunity to create a new narrative from brief disjointed experiences and for others to contribute too. Widening the frame and extending the conversation were also key factors in creating opportunities – and the space – for a different perspective and change with stuck or puzzling cases. Team colleagues increasingly contributed to this new narrative which became shared by the whole team rather than the consultee alone. This extended conversation and synthesis, commented on by Launer

(2002), may be particularly helpful where the practitioner has a disjointed or very partial view of the patient.

The style of consultation during the initial explorative phase and the second phase that succeeded it shared much with what Page and Woskett (1994) describe as a 'cyclical' model. In this there is a focus on facilitating the individual to enhance and fully utilise their own skills and knowledge supported by an explicit process of review and evaluation. During this period the focus of consultation was, nonetheless, largely on single case presentations, although this evolved too. Initially, the process was more akin to individual consultation in a group, whereas this rapidly developed as group members were actively encouraged to participate and contribute too.

---

**Case study 1.6**

Natasha was 18 years old and living with her sister when she disclosed to one of the newer GPs in the practice that her father had been sexually abusing her. The team consultation revealed a fuller picture of Natasha, who was notorious for her difficult behaviour and had a significant history of minor injury. It now seemed likely that the injuries, often accompanied by failure to heal, resulted both from assault and from self-harm, the latter only becoming apparent shortly before, after a pen became lodged in a dental bridge which had been repeatedly refitted following an assault.

Natasha was one of three offspring in a family that made substantial and inappropriate demands on the primary care team. One example of the latter was when, responding to a Christmas Day home visit, the on-call doctor was met by naked carousers but no significant health threat. Natasha's mother had been described as 'ineffective' but had withdrawn from support, her father chronically disabled, her brother alcoholic, whilst her sister was known to be prostituting herself in the neighbourhood. Living with her sister might provide an escape but carried its own risks.

It is not surprising that 'de-listing' this family and Natasha herself had at least been discussed and the family were a focus of significant anger for the practice team and others. Both the family context and Natasha's own history made it difficult to hear her concerns and identify a course of action. The consultation workshop helped to elucidate the individual and family circumstances and enabled the team to share their feelings of anger and frustration before focusing on an attempt to understand Natasha's experience and needs. A new 'narrative' was created which included a realisation that Natasha's behaviour had much to do with the assault, abuse and neglect that she had experienced and that she may now be asking for help to change her life.

The practice team retained Natasha on the practice list and devised a strategy for managing her healthcare amongst the team. It was agreed to discuss with Natasha the options of rehousing away from her sister, referral for mental health assessment and counselling. Subsequently, each of these options was successfully taken advantage of by Natasha who 'settled' to some extent despite her history. A few years later, having moved away, Natasha returned to the practice to say 'thank you'.

The second and third phases of the consultation workshop were punctuated by significant departures and arrivals in the team. New practice partners were dragooned into joining the workshop and did so tentatively at first: the multi-disciplinary contextual approach was by now well established as newcomers reported that it took some time to understand the cases being presented with their complex histories and extended ramifications. Conversely they reported that the workshop was a good introduction to the practice, their new multidisciplinary colleagues and their roles.

## A mature group: co-consultation

In the third phase, the workshop evolved into a style of consultation that had more in common with Proctor and Inskipp's type 3 model of group supervision (ibid.). In this the focus is initially with the individual presenting the case – although it became more common that shared presentations were made – but the consultant would also encourage other members to participate, not only provid-ing information about the case as before, but also with challenges or suggestions for a new understanding drawn from their own knowledge of the case or their professional skills. In this style of consultation, the consultant facilitated the group in sharing responsibility for the tasks of group consultation.

More uniquely, as this was a multidisciplinary work team, the consultation included the existing or potential involvement of other team members in responding to the case. In this phase of the workshop the consultant's own skills and knowledge were also brought into play more, but merely as one perspective or skill set within the workshop. As the consultation workshop was interrupted (due to the consultant moving away), it seemed that a fourth evolutionary phase might have begun: this could be described as 'facilitation of co-consultation'. In this model rather than 'peer consultation', the chairing and facilitation of the consultant remains an important contribution but increasingly the participants determine the content and process of the sessions, deploying the group manners and skills they have honed over preceding sessions.

## Concluding remarks

It remained somewhat puzzling that this apparently successful initiative was not replicated with other practice teams. The initiative was known of in the local general practice community but neither practice nor consultant proselytised for the workshop, and although a number of tentative requests were made to replicate the workshop, these did not come to fruition. This may be because such teams lacked some of the essential foundations: an internal champion, a sound team 'dynamic' (illustrated at least by pre-existing and effective team meetings), a commitment to learning together and a sense that it was 'safe enough' to share one's more troubling cases. This seemed to reflect the situation of one 'leaver' whilst a second leaver reported that although she had found the workshop helpful – in much the same way as other participants – her new role was much less pressured and stressful and so such an exercise would not seem so worthwhile.

As the NHS has again become preoccupied with a limited set of performance targets, it is also noteworthy that this consultation workshop was first initiated at a time when formal financial contracting was taking off in the NHS. Early NHS contracting was organised solely in relation to direct patient contact with no ready scope for an initiative like this. The context then was a consultant already fully occupied and with the activity and outcomes of this initiative lying outside the performance indicators defined by an NHS newly preoccupied with performance measurement and management. The practice, however, became convinced that this consultation was cost-effective for them and, later as belated converts to GP fund-holding and as a PMS pilot, insisted that they would find a way to formally contract for the service if necessary.

We have become much more aware in CAMHS, in particular, of the benefits to be gained from more active relationships between primary and secondary specialist healthcare. As primary mental health workers are deployed to support primary care with consultation and advice as well as brief interventions, we need to ensure that the processes of contracting, commissioning and performance management do not inhibit such initiatives but rather capture their spirit and support them.

This consultation workshop worked well for its participants and was favourably evaluated by them for its contribution to learning, clinical practice and team development. Although not formulated or discussed in such terms, this was also, and undoubtedly, a 'peer review' contribution to the clinical governance agenda. The initiative described here was very much driven by primary care: this is illustrated in part through the range of ages and presenting problems in the consultation workshop. This driver is also demonstrated in the style of the workshop and its emphasis on consultation that facilitated, focused and enhanced the existing skills and knowledge of the participants. The workshop exploited the psychological and relationship skills of the consultant and was not designed to deliver psychological or relationship 'therapies', but it did bring to bear an enhanced understanding of behaviour in the consulting room, in families and in the local community and healthcare systems. Nonetheless, even in a more flexible performance management environment it might be easy to overlook the human and team factors that contributed to this consultation workshop's success.

---

### Learning points

Key learning points which contributed to the workshop's effectiveness were:

*Team learning points*
- A team commitment to working and learning together
- The value of a respected champion helping to support, organise and contribute to the workshop
- Organisational support in protected time, space and sustenance
- A degree of comfort with each other and the courage to share difficulties at times of personal and professional uncertainty
- The opportunity to 'test the water' and explicitly review and re-contract

*Consultant learning points*
- Explicit respect for the different skills and knowledge of team members

*Continued*

- An inclusive approach with an emphasis on safety and supportive challenge
- Consultation skills – particularly those drawn from systemic practice
- Expertise in human behaviour and relationships
- A focus which has its origin in primary care rather than any rigid delimitations of specialist secondary healthcare (e.g. children, mental health)

*Learning points for the process of working together*
- The creation of safety, mutual respect and 'good group manners'
- A supportive, validating approach
- Clear focus and clarity about the task or question being asked
- Structure for the case consultation
- Recognition of the evolving style of the workshop.

## References

Caplan G (1970) *The Theory and Practice of Mental Health Consultation.* Tavistock, London.

Launer J (2002) *Narrative-Based Primary Care: a practical guide.* Radcliffe Medical Press, Oxford.

Page S and Woskett V (1994) *Supervising the Counsellor: a cyclical model.* Routledge, London.

Proctor B and Inskipp F (2001) Group supervision. In: Scaife JM (2001) *Supervision in the Mental Health Professions: a practitioner's guide.* Brunner-Routledge, Hove, East Sussex.

Rosenblatt A and Mayer JE (1975) Objectionable supervisory styles: students' views. *Social Work.* **May:** 184–9.

## Further reading

Hawkins P and Shohet R (1989) *Supervision in the Helping Professions.* Open University Press, Milton Keynes.

Inskipp F and Proctor B (1988) *Skills for Supervising and Being Supervised.* Cascade Publications, Twickenham, Middlesex.

Inskipp F and Proctor B (1994) *Making the Most of Supervision: Part 2.* Cascade Publications, Twickenham, Middlesex.

McDaniel SH, Wynne LC and Weber TT (1986) The territory of systems consultation. In: Wynne CW, McDaniel SH and Weber TT (eds) *Systems Consultation: a new perspective for family therapy.* Guilford Press, New York.

Scaife JM (2001) *Supervision in the Mental Health Professions: a practitioner's guide.* Brunner-Routledge, Hove, East Sussex.

Steinberg D (1989) *Interprofessional Consultation.* Blackwell, Oxford.

# Chapter 2

# Child mental health consultation in primary care: the developing role of the primary mental health worker

*Fiona Gale*

## Introduction

The demand for child and adolescent mental health services (CAMHS) has escalated during the last decade. Such a rise in demand has emerged from an increased recognition of mental health need amongst children (Kurtz 1994) and changing patterns of service provision in several sectors (Kurtz *et al.* 1994). As a result of such changes, community CAMHS teams have accumulated longer waiting times, with a reduction in responsiveness (Health Advisory Service [HAS] 1995). Emerging problems are now being increasingly identified and managed within those services that have first contact with children on a day-to-day basis.

The publication of the 'Emerging Findings' document for the National Service Framework for Children (Department of Health [DoH] 2003) emphasised the need to ensure that the CAMHS workforce at all levels of provision, including universal services for children, is skilled and competent in meeting the needs of its population. This requires a workforce that is trained to deliver a full range of interventions, including comprehensive mental health assessment and a variety of treatments, based on best available evidence. The importance of training and support for universal services is also highlighted within the document. The development of such a skilled workforce in universal CAMHS requires collaboration between specialist CAMHS and front-line professionals to develop creative ways of enhancing and supporting the workforce (Gale 2003). The 'Emerging Findings' report also suggests the template for comprehensive CAMHS, which includes mental health promotion, early intervention and enhancement of capacity at tier 1.

Front-line professionals working with children and young people on a day-to-day basis can frequently encounter early presentations of mental health difficulties, which can fall anywhere along the continuum. The prevalence of children experiencing mental health problems in primary care has been found to be between 20–25% (Kramer and Garralda 2000). Whilst some of these problems are complex and require referral to specialist CAMHS, others can be successfully managed within universal services, with ongoing support from specialist colleagues.

## Recommendations from key publications

Both the report 'Together We Stand' (HAS 1995), a thematic review of CAMHS in England and Wales, and the 'Emerging Findings' make key recommendations for agencies to work in collaboration to provide a co-ordinated, strategic response to the commissioning and delivery of CAMHS. They also suggest that specialist services should develop more consultative ways of working and enhance their support for tier 1 professionals, who remain largely unsupported in their work with children and young people.

In 1995, 'Together We Stand' introduced the role of the CAMHS primary mental health worker (PMHW), located within specialist CAMHS provision (tier 2/3), working at the interface with universal services. These recommendations were also affirmed by reports from the House of Commons Health Committee (DoH 1997), the Mental Health Foundation (1999) and the Audit Commission (2000) and consolidated within the 'Emerging Findings' report. Such policies have influenced the escalation of investment in the recruitment of PMHWs and development of the PMHW role across the United Kingdom (UK).

## The primary mental health worker role in CAMHS

The main emphasis of the PMHW role is to strengthen and support the provision of CAMHS within universal services by building capacity and capability in relation to early identification and intervention regarding children's mental health need, thereby closing the gap between universal services and specialist CAMHS. Responsive provision may therefore be planned according to the levels of identified mental health need. Such support enables professionals within universal services to effectively recognise children's mental health strengths and difficulties. It also offers opportunities to improve interagency collaboration in the provision of CAMHS and provides accessible intervention for children and families within a non-stigmatising environment. Active promotion of mental health in children and their families can also be achieved by offering a needs-led service in the community, through formalised support and joint work in partnership with front-line professionals.

The PMHW provides this support through a combination of advice, consultation, supervision, training, liaison and joint working. The PMHW role also includes assessment and intervention with children and young people and the facilitation of access to specialist CAMHS for those children and young people who require that level of intervention. The principle of joint working and planning with other agencies and services, whilst encouraging further development of existing skills in recognising and managing child mental health, also encourages a universal ownership of children's mental health by all professionals. In turn, this enables specialist CAMHS to maximise their efficiency by targeting need appropriate to their skills and expertise.

## The context of primary mental health work

Professionals undertaking the PMHW role can be from a variety of professional backgrounds. It is important that they have significant experience of working with children, including those with mental health needs, as well as a broad range of skills in diverse clinical and behavioural presentations. They should also be able to make comprehensive assessments of the child's level of mental health need and be experienced in a range of therapeutic interventions.

PMHWs are usually allocated to a community CAMHS team, or work within a specific CAMHS context. For example, they can target particularly vulnerable or hard to reach groups of children and young people, such as those with a disability, looked-after children, young offenders, homeless young people or black and minority ethnic groups. Being allocated to a defined population enables the PMHW to become involved in detailed collaboration with professionals who relate to that community, therefore developing an understanding and relationship with that population, thus enabling the creation of a needs-led service.

## The developing role

Since 1995 there has been a rapid growth in developments around the UK. There are a number of emerging models.

### Single PMHWs

These dedicated PMHW posts located within specialist CAMHS offer some components of the role (i.e. consultation, training and liaison) to a large population of professionals or all aspects of the role to a smaller locality or defined population. The drawback with such posts is that workers can become very isolated when working out in the community; therefore it is very important for them to have clear supervision frameworks and regular contact with other PMHW peers.

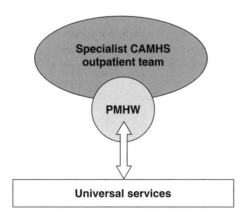

Figure 2.1 Single primary mental health worker model.

### Liaison-attachment models

Here the PMHW is located within a specific service or agency, i.e. in schools, particularly within some of the multi-agency behaviour and education support teams (BEST), within a health centre or general practitioner (GP) practice or within social services. This model is similar to some of those being adopted in adult mental health within the Common Mental Health Problems initiatives (DoH 2002). Some models tend to offer direct work as well as consultation and joint work (Neira-Munoz and Ward 1998); however, they need to establish clear pathways to specialist CAMHS to ensure that those children whose level of need requires a higher level of intervention are able to access services in a timely manner.

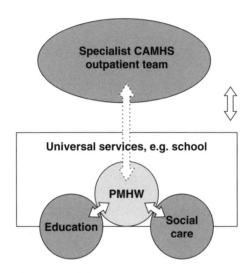

**Figure 2.2** Liaison-attachment model.

## Consultation and liaison services

Consultation and liaison services are usually provided by the PMHW through an individual worker or a small team. The role can be also developed as part of an existing post (i.e. a children's social worker, community psychiatric nurse or specialist teacher) or as part of a secondment into specialist CAMHS. The model includes support, consultation and liaison to front-line professionals. Access can be directly to the individual/team or through specialist CAMHS. Particular aspects of the role may be offered as time can be limited and target populations large. The focus here is on building on existing capacity and resources within tier 1 in order to meet children's mental health needs.

## Multi-agency or community CAMH initiatives

Child mental health services have also been developed and operate in the community on a parallel with universal services (tier 1). These initiatives have a range of child mental health workers, including PMHWs, working within defined localities or communities and are based in local infrastructures such as primary schools, children's centres, health centres or general practice surgeries. Some teams operate as independent services with their own referral systems. The

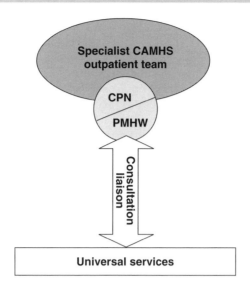

Figure 2.3 Consultation–liaison model.

workers within such services are linked primarily to that community, rather than with the tier 2 CAMHS, although there are often agreed links to specialist tiers for those children with identified levels of need that meet the criteria for such intervention (Appleton and Hammond-Rowley 2000). Such teams tend to offer a higher proportion of early intervention with children and families, as well as enhancing existing universal resources.

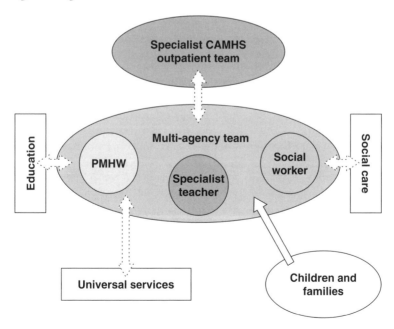

Figure 2.4 Community CAMHS initiatives.

## Primary mental health worker teams

These are large teams of PMHWs located within tier 2/3 CAMHS, offering all components of the role to professionals, children and families in primary care (Arcelus *et al.* 2001). More recently there have been developments with looked-after children and within youth offending teams.

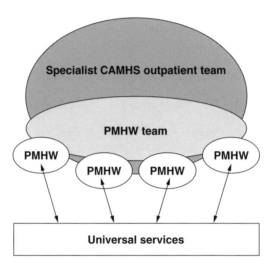

**Figure 2.5** Primary mental health worker teams located in CAMHS.

---

**Case study 2.1 The Leicestershire CAMHS Primary Mental Health Team**

The Leicestershire Primary Mental Health Team consists of a large number of PMHWs, several of whom work to specific target areas in the community, and others based within the youth offending teams (YOTs) and looked-after children services (LACs). The team is located within tier 2/3 CAMHS, with the PMHW relating to the corresponding community outpatient team in CAMHS, as well as being a member of the primary mental health team. The team is structured so that leadership, overall clinical supervision, strategic/operational development and co-ordination of the team are provided by a PMHW Head of Service, with senior PMHWs providing some clinical supervision/managerial support to their colleagues. As well as relating to particular fields or areas, the PMHWs work very much as a team, therefore enabling a sharing of skills and knowledge across boundaries. In addition, the community PMHWs link in with multi-agency, community-based child behaviour intervention initiatives (CBIIs). The CBIIs are one of 24 CAMHS innovations projects being overseen by Young Minds and the Department of Health.

Target populations

The Leicestershire Primary Mental Health Team covers inner-city, semi-urban and rural areas of a general population of approximately 900 000 across three local authorities. The community PMHWs operate within identified target localities of approximately 50 000–60 000 population (or 11 000 children); however, the population figure has been found to vary dependent on the needs of the population – for example, in inner-city areas, where the need is greatest. PMHWs tend to focus on a population of around 25 000, whereas in semi-urban or rural areas the population can be greater. These areas would also be dependent on the other services available to the community. The PMHWs for young offenders and looked-after children work across the whole CAMHS population in relation to these vulnerable groups (Callaghan *et al.* 2002).

# The Leicestershire model of primary mental health work

The PMHW model developed in Leicester is an integrated approach based on a combination of biological, psychological and sociological theories, which complement the range of backgrounds and experience of PMHWs. The process, which is centred around three levels of intervention, has been developed from research relating to primary care professionals' experience of the PMHW role (Gale 1999, 2004; Gale and Vostanis 2003), from mental health consultation (Caplan 1970) and from consultation–liaison models in adult psychiatry, mental health nursing and within the helping professions (Roberts 1997; Tunmore 1997; Hawkins and Shohet 2000). Each level can prompt a move to another level, and there can be an interface with other agencies or specialist CAMHS at any stage, dependent on the determined level of need. The process starts in all instances with consultation.

Consultation may reveal a need for training, ongoing consultation or supervision, or may progress to joint working with the referring professional or an identified professional deemed more appropriate to meet the child's needs. It may also lead to liaison with other agencies, or in some instances to assessment and direct intervention with children and families. Consultation can also identify those children presenting with more severe mental health difficulties requiring specialist CAMHS intervention (Arcelus *et al.* 2002).

The PMHW actively filters referrals to the CAMHS community teams through their referral meeting or through direct requests for consultation by professionals in universal services or the CBIIs. The model enables both the PMHW and primary care professionals to define the level of support and intervention required. Such an approach is necessary to achieve shared goals, i.e. managing the child's mental health needs successfully in tier 1 or ensuring access to the service appropriate to the determined level of mental health need.

# First-level intervention: consultation, supervision and training consultation

PMHWs offer consultation as part of their 'first level' of interventions, which includes supervision and training. Before describing the consultation process in

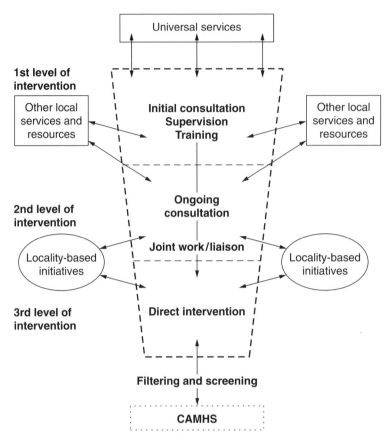

**1st level of intervention**

**2nd level of intervention**

**3rd level of intervention**

Universal services

Other local services and resources

Initial consultation
Supervision
Training

Other local services and resources

Ongoing consultation

Locality-based initiatives

Joint work/liaison

Locality-based initiatives

Direct intervention

**Filtering and screening**

**CAMHS**

**Figure 2.6** Models of service delivery: primary mental health worker (Gale 1999; Gale and Vostanis 2003).

more detail, it is useful to consider briefly these other first-level interventions, along with the relationships that link them.

## Supervision

Supervision differs from consultation in that it is primarily educative. The aim is to improve the ability of tier 1 professionals to manage child mental health needs more effectively by improving their skill and knowledge base, thus enabling more effective practice (Regel and Davies 1995). Supervision can take the form of individual or group support and can also act as a means of consolidating multi-agency training offered by PMHWs. This component of the role should neither replace nor conflict with the professionals' own clinical supervision.

As an example, in Leicestershire the PMHWs have been involved in a project to train teachers in anger management techniques for use in the classroom and to provide them with specific ongoing supervision to enable them to apply it to their practice.

## Training

Regular multi-agency training programmes offered to tier 1 professionals can increase and build upon understanding of children's mental health issues and can consolidate their existing knowledge through experiential learning (Sebuliba and Vostanis 2001). It should not seek to turn front-line staff into specialists in children's mental health, but rather enable them to recognise and manage child mental health problems at an early stage. By providing training on a multi-agency basis, professionals can develop a knowledge and shared ownership of children's mental health, and develop a broad knowledge base and a theoretical framework to make informed choices on the best care pathways for children's individual needs (Dogra *et al.* 2002).

# The primary mental health worker and consultation

Within the PMHW role definition, consultation can vary according to the context in which it is undertaken. The aims of consultation are to jointly define the child's mental health needs, to consider the most appropriate ways of meeting them and to enable the building of capacity and knowledge within primary care. The consultation framework enables professionals to challenge their own practice and to consider alternatives to managing children's mental health needs.

The principles of consultation within the PMHW role have been drawn from work on mental health consultation and have parallels with consultation/liaison psychiatry (Caplan 1970). The liaison psychiatry role was developed in the USA to make the best use of limited psychiatric resources in the community and was also undertaken by psychiatrists in the UK in the general medical setting (Lipowski 1968 and 1981; Roberts 1997), i.e. when patients who had resorted to deliberate self-harm presented to accident and emergency departments. Access to such a consultation resource is considered to be essential in collaboration with primary care professionals and aids in the management of psychological problems and decision making about treatment directions for children (Leonard *et al.* 1990). Consultation is a central tenet of the PMHW role (Hobbs and Murray 1999; Appleton and Hammond-Rowley 2000) and vital in the initiation of integrated multi-agency practice.

Within the Leicestershire model, consultation is seen as a collaborative relationship. The consultant (PMHW) is defined as having specialist CAMH expertise and works indirectly on a problem or dilemma with the consultee (tier 1 practitioner). Within this partnership, the consultee is defined as a competent autonomous practitioner who may accept or reject advice (Caplan 1970; Tunmore 1997). Consultation may be considered to be supportive, normative or formative (Caplan 1970; Tunmore 1997). Within this exercise the consulting professionals retain clinical responsibility within their own professional guidelines.

Consultation has been developed within the PMHW role in a variety of formats and is viewed as being on a continuum, with different levels that relate closely to Caplan's (1970) classification of consultation. This ranges from telephone advice and support, which is the most commonly utilised aspect of consultation, to advanced face-to-face consultation or regular consultation/supervision groups. Regular group consultations can also be run on a multi-agency or uniprofessional basis, such as with health visitors, community paediatricians and within GP surgeries. It can also be useful for PMHWs to provide advice and consultation to local community forums and voluntary agencies as these professionals regularly encounter children's mental health problems. Some of these agencies can come across mental health problems which can be of a more severe nature, often where families have not wanted to access mental health services because of perceptions of stigma. It is important that consultation takes place within a wider service framework as consultants will require access to information and resources that can be shared with consulting professionals.

The initial part of the consultative process always begins with the PMHW providing consultation to primary care professionals in the form of telephone and face-to-face consultation. This initial consultation is usually accessed when a professional has concerns about a child's mental well-being, is unsure where to refer or what services are available, or when a case has already been referred to the community CAMHS team and allocated to the PMHW.

Following a preliminary discussion, it is often apparent that the primary care professional could manage the case effectively with support from the PMHW. At this point, there is an agreement between the two professionals that leads to a more advanced stage of consultation. This would involve the development of a written contract surrounding the consultation, which would identify aims and desired outcomes for the consultation session and look at the process for a supportive relationship.

At this stage of consultation the PMHWs use a screening tool to determine the child's level of need. The screening tool is based on a comprehensive mental health assessment (Dogra *et al.* 2002). The session would ask specific questions of the consultee in relation to different aspects of the child's presentation, in order to establish the level of child mental health concern. The tool also provides a focus for the consultation and aids in identifying the appropriate tier of CAMHS required, thus having the function of early recognition of mental health problems. For example, screening a child defined as presenting with a risk of self-harm would then immediately indicate the need to consider intervention by specialist CAMHS.

The child mental health screening tool is shown in Box 2.1.

---

**Box 2.1 Establishing the level of child mental health concern** (Dogra *et al.* 2002)

- Describe the concern in detail – getting examples of specific events or incidents.
- When did the concern start? (onset)
- How long has it been going on? (duration)
- How often does it happen? (frequency)
- Is the situation getting worse/remaining the same/getting better?
- What actions have been taken to address the concerns? What has worked so far? (parents/carers and practitioners)
- Are there ongoing medical investigations?
- How is the concern affecting the young person? (impact)

Any screening tool intended for self-completion by front-line professionals prior to consultation would need to be accompanied by a programme of training. Consultation within the PMHW role is on a continuum ranging from telephone advice and support to advanced face-to-face consultation, where the PMHW and the primary care professional meet regularly to agree goals and review work.

In more advanced consultation, the consultee still retains responsibility for the case and can decide how they utilise the decisions made during the consultation. The role of the consultant would continue to be an enabling activity, which encourages and advises the consultee in relation to their work with the child and their decision making. Within this process there is also the provision for a follow-up meeting to review work. It must be acknowledged that consultation does not replace the consultee's own clinical supervision; therefore, it is important to reflect this in the contract when developing it.

## Elements of the consultation process

The PMHW must be able to provide a facilitative role, in which the context of the dilemma is widened and a theoretical framework can be presented which guides the enquiry. The framework used can be from a range of theoretical perspectives, e.g. solution-focused, motivational or systemic consultation. Throughout the consultation there will be assessment of the nature of need and the consultant must have sufficient knowledge about child mental health, therapeutic interventions and also service provision available, including the role of specialist CAMHS.

The advanced consultation process should also identify monitoring and review arrangement for the case so that the needs of the child can be reassessed if necessary and the approach adjusted accordingly. In Leicestershire, consultation is recorded using a pro forma with sections for outcomes and review dates. A copy is always sent to the consultee for their records as they continue to have clinical responsibility for the case at this stage.

## Messages from research

Research which examined primary care professionals' perceptions and experience of the PMHW role (Gale 1999) indicated that they valued a combination of consultation, training and supervision, followed by joint working and liaison. A total of 79.3% indicated consultation was of most value to them and 58.4% felt they had been able to tackle children's mental health difficulties, during the first year, with support and training from the PMHW. Tier 1 professionals considered the PMHW role to enable an unprecedented access to CAMHS and was a valuable resource in helping them manage children's mental health problems. During a recent evaluation of the Leicestershire consultation model, 68% of professionals accessing consultation with a PMHW felt that their confidence had improved in relation to dealing with children's mental health problems.

## Consultation in practice: the use of solution-focused models

In Leicestershire, the consultation process has been further developed using solution-focused approaches (*see* Chapter 4). A group of health visitors have undertaken training in the use of solution-focused brief therapy (de Shazer 1985; George *et al.* 1999) and were offered ongoing support and consultation on specific cases by the PMHWs. The solution-focused approach fits well with the ethos behind child mental health consultation in primary care as it seeks to build on strengths and capacities (George *et al.* 2001).

## When consultation is not enough

Second- and third-level interventions may follow consultation. These include liaison, joint working and (at level three) direct intervention. Joint work between primary care professionals and PMHWs is agreed and negotiated through the process of consultation. It is a two-way learning activity, in that both professionals set agreed aims and objectives for the intervention. Once the joint working process has ended, supportive, consultative or supervisory plans are agreed with the practitioner working with the child, thus enabling ongoing communication and management. Examples of these are given in Box 2.2.

---

**Box 2.2 Joint work negotiated through consultation**

- Support for the practitioner in the work they are already undertaking, assisting them in developing choices for intervention
- Joint assessment with a practitioner already involved in a case, for the purpose of understanding the child's or the family's needs in relation to mental health
- Training and support about the child mental health assessment process or a specific management/intervention technique
- Development of jointly facilitated groups in the community for young people and parents

---

## Third-level direct intervention with children and families

Third-level interventions are defined as those requiring direct intervention. At any stage of the model it may be necessary for the PMHW to undertake direct intervention with children and families in cases where:

- mental health difficulties have not been responsive to methods and interventions undertaken by tier 1 professionals
- the level of need is not appropriate for intervention within specialist CAMHS.

Direct interventions should be brief and tailored to the child's and family's identified needs. The child must also be suitable for management by primary care professionals, once the intervention is complete (Davis *et al.* 1997). In such cases, the PMHW will offer a brief focused intervention, followed by a formal review with the child, the family and, where possible, primary care professionals involved. Direct work should be evidence based and drawn from a range of interventions, for example cognitive behavioural therapy or solution-focused brief therapy. It can also include the provision of target group work programmes.

## Challenges in implementing a PMHW consultation model in primary care

Although some specialist or community CAMHS practitioners have traditionally offered consultation to other agencies and many CAMHS have existing liaison schemes, the introduction of the PMHW role has increased the emphasis on the value of consultation in preventing children's mental health problems and working in partnership to tackle children's mental health problems at a primary level (Dogra *et al.* 2002; Gale and Vostanis 2003). Successful examples of other models include the Solihull Approach, focusing on supporting parenting in the community through a combination of consultation, counselling and training (Douglas and Ginty 2001); others have developed specialist health visitors to work on supporting parents whose children have emotional or behaviour problems (e.g. Davies *et al.* 1997; Day *et al.* 1998).

## Future focus

It is vital that PMHWs also have knowledge and experience in tier 2/3 (i.e. specialist) CAMHS work to enable them to facilitate the consultative process. Links with the specialist CAMH team are also crucial to ensure that the interface between non-specialist and specialist CAMHS is successful when children's mental health needs, identified during the consultation process, require intervention at the next level. Clinical supervision for PMHWs should be available both within the framework of the multidisciplinary team and from within their own field.

Although there are different models of primary mental health work emerging throughout the UK, it is becoming apparent that the support of CAMHS through effective tier 1 working is paramount. With the introduction of the PMHW role having a principal focus on reducing waiting lists for specialist CAMHS and the aim to work collaboratively with primary care, it is imperative that the consultation, training and joint working elements of the role are given priority. Without this, it can prove difficult to provide the interface between tiers and to build and support capacity within primary care. As a result the PMHW role can become a satellite service with all similar problems to specialist CAMHS and primary care professionals can develop unrealistic expectations.

The PMHW role can be seen as a controversial approach to meeting the mental health needs of children as it often challenges professionals' preconceptions about responsibilities for CAMH service provision. The consultation aspect of the role can sometimes be seen as denying access to specialist services or 'gate-keeping', which could potentially cause frustrations and alienation. One solution is to ensure the initial service planning and development includes potential users, which in this case would include tier 1 professionals.

Involving professionals at an early stage in the development of the PMHW model helps to promote collaboration and understanding. The challenge of engaging professionals in collaborative working and of understanding the CAMHS agenda is an integral component of the PMHW role as new colleagues begin and new pressures in tier 1 emerge. Some professional groups within primary care can be reluctant to use the consultation process as their time and capacity to liaise is limited. It is therefore important to have an understanding of their needs and to be creative in offering consultation. The PMHW also needs to be proactive in working with professionals and community leaders representing vulnerable or excluded groups in the community to establish appropriate ways of providing a supportive consultation service.

# References

Appleton PL and Hammond-Rowley S (2000) Addressing the population burden of child and adolescent mental health problems: a primary care model. *Child Psychology and Psychiatry Review.* **5**: 9–16.

Arcelus J, Gale F and Vostanis P (2001) Characteristics of children and parents attending a primary mental health service. *European Child and Adolescent Psychiatry Newsletter.* **10** (1): 91–5.

Arcelus J, Gale F and Vostanis P (2002) Child mental health problems in primary care. In: Nolan P and Badger F (eds) *Promoting Collaboration in Primary Mental Health Care.* Nelson Thornes, London.

Audit Commission (2000) *With Children in Mind: child and adolescent mental health services.* Audit Commission Publications, Oxford.

Callaghan J, Young B and Vostanis P (2002) *Primary Mental Health Workers within Youth Offending Teams: evaluation of a new service model.* University of Leicester, Leicester.

Caplan G (1970) *The Theory and Practice of Mental Health Consultation.* Tavistock, London.

Davis H, Spurr P, Cox A *et al.* (1997) A description and evaluation of a community child mental health service. *Clinical Child Psychology and Psychiatry.* **2**: 221–38.

Day C, Davis H and Hind R (1998) The development of a community child and family mental health service. *Child Care, Health and Development.* **24** (6): 487–500.

de Shazer S (1985) *Keys to Solution in Brief Therapy.* Norton Press, New York.

Department of Health (1997) *Developing Partnerships in Mental Health.* HMSO, London.

Department of Health (2002) *Fast-forwarding Primary Care Mental Health: 'gateway' workers.* HMSO, London.

Department of Health (2003) *Getting the Right Start: the National Service Framework for Children, Young People and Maternity Services – emerging findings.* HMSO, London.

Dogra N, Parkin A, Gale F *et al.* (2002) *A Multi-disciplinary Handbook of Child and Adolescent Mental Health for Front-line Professionals.* Jessica Kingsley Publishers, London.

Douglas H and Ginty M (2001) The Solihull Approach: changes in health-visiting practice. (A systematic approach to working with children with behaviour problems.) *Community Practitioner.* **74** (6): 222–4.

Gale FJ (1999) When tiers are not enough: an evaluation of the perceptions and experiences amongst primary care professionals of the primary mental health worker role within CAMHS. Unpublished MA Thesis in Research Methodology. University of Central England, Birmingham.

Gale F (2003) Working towards a comprehensive CAMHS: child and adolescent mental health – the next three years. *Child and Adolescent Mental Health in Primary Care.* **1** (3): 72–6.

Gale F (2004) *Interim Report on the Training Needs of Child Mental Health Workers (Primary Mental Health Workers) in CAMHS.* National CAMHS Support Service, Leicestershire,

Northamptonshire and Rutland Strategic Health Authority. (Available from www.camhs.org.)

Gale F and Vostanis P (2003) The primary mental health worker in child and adolescent mental health services. *Clinical Child Psychology and Psychiatry.* **8** (2): 227–40.

George E, Iverson C and Ratner H (1999) *Problem to Solution: brief therapy with individuals and families* (revised and expanded edition). Brief Therapy Practice, London.

George E, Iverson C and Ratner H (2001) *Supervision and Consultation: a solution-focused approach.* BT Press, London.

Hawkins D and Shohet R (2000) *Supervision in the Helping Professions.* Open University Press, Buckingham.

Health Advisory Service (1995) *Together We Stand: the commissioning, role and management of child and adolescent mental health services.* HMSO, London.

Hobbs R and Murray ET (1999) Specialist Liaison Nurses. *BMJ.* **318**: 683–4.

Kramer T and Garralda EM (2000) Child and adolescent mental health problems in primary care. *Advances in Psychiatric Treatment.* **6**: 287–94.

Kurtz Z (1994) *Treating Children Well: a guide to using the evidence base in commissioning and managing for the mental health of children and young people.* Mental Health Foundation, London.

Kurtz Z, Thornes R and Wolkind S (1994) *Services for the Mental Health of Children and Young People in England: a national review.* South Thames Regional Health Authority, London.

Leonard I, Babbs C and Freed FH (1990) Psychiatric referrals within the hospital: the communication process. *Journal of Research in Social Medicine.* **83**: 241–4.

Lipowski ZJ (1968) Review of consultation psychiatry and psychosomatic medicine. III: thematic issues. *Psychosomatic Medicine.* **33**: 395–422.

Lipowski ZJ (1981) Liaison psychiatry, liaison nursing and behavioural medicine. *Comprehensive Psychiatry.* **148**: 194–7.

Mental Health Foundation (1999) *Bright Futures: promoting children and young people's mental health.* Mental Health Foundation, London.

Neira-Munoz E and Ward D (1998) Side by side. *Health Services Journal.* **13 August**: 26–7.

Regel S and Davies J (1995) The future of mental health nurses in liaison psychiatry. *British Journal of Nursing.* **4** (18): 1052–6.

Roberts D (1997) Liaison mental health nursing: origins, definition and prospects. *Journal of Advanced Nursing.* **25**: 101–8.

Sebuliba D and Vostanis P (2001) Child and adolescent mental health training from primary care staff. *Clinical Child Psychology and Psychiatry.* **6**: 191–204.

Tunmore R (1997) Mental health liaison and consultation. *Nursing Standard.* **11** (50): 46–51.

Chapter 3

# A psychodynamic approach to consultation within two contrasting school settings

*Louise Emanuel*

## Introduction

This chapter describes consultation to two different schools over several years by a psychoanalytically trained child psychotherapist. In the first example consultation meetings were provided to the staff of a school for children with severe learning disabilities, whilst in the second the focus was on staff consultation and brief interventions with pupils and their parents. The setting for this was a fee-paying, high-achieving school.

The term 'consultation' implies discussion with professionals within an organisation to help them think about aspects of their work setting, as well as individual children and families about whom they may feel concerned. The aim of the consultation is to facilitate detailed consideration of issues arising for staff in relation to their teaching role and concerning children in their professional care. Through this process a different perspective on a situation is offered that might help develop strategies for change. It does not include direct clinical work with the client group.

As the consultant is a psychoanalytically trained child psychotherapist, the framework for thinking about institutional dynamics involves an understanding of unconscious processes and key psychoanalytic concepts and is informed by clinical work with young children, adolescents and families. One focus of this chapter will therefore be the application of some of the tools for understanding individuals in a psychotherapeutic context to an understanding of institutional dynamics.

The author describes how children who have learning difficulties may protect themselves from the pain of 'not knowing' by devaluing (or rubbishing) the role of the teacher as someone promoting creative mental activity. This can lead to teachers feeling deskilled and can have implications for staff management and team structure. Case examples illustrate these points. The second part of the chapter describes the author's work in a school for more able children, and how consultation with staff and brief therapeutic work with students with emotional difficulties enabled positive changes to take place.

# Consultation to a school for children with severe learning disabilities

Consultation work to this school is described in the form of teacher discussion groups and consultations to the senior management team to try and illustrate how a psychoanalytic understanding of unconscious processes operating within the school may help to facilitate beneficial changes, which impact on relationships at all levels.

## Early damage

Staff in this kind of school care for damaged, often emotionally disturbed children. The unconscious projections from children into teaching staff, and from teaching staff into the senior staff team, can be felt to be overwhelming unless help is offered to think about them (*see* Box 3.1).

---

**Box 3.1  Concept of splitting and projection**

This unconscious process involves the fantasy of separating off some (usually) undesirable aspects of the self, or painful/unpleasant emotional states, distancing oneself from these traits or feelings by getting rid of them out of the self into another person. (This is, for example, the basis of scapegoating.)

---

As the consultant has heard details of the increasing number of physically and mentally damaged children who also display serious levels of emotional disturbance, she has begun to think that the troubled behaviour and interactions described by staff may reflect a disturbance which occurred in the early relationship between mother (or primary carer) and baby, a kind of 'mismatch' between them and a disruption of the normal bonding process. This may partly be connected to the impact on the mother of the news that her baby is damaged in some way, which may then interfere with her capacity to provide containment for her child.

Central to understanding of the role of a well-functioning organisation (family/parental couple, etc.) is the psychoanalyst Wilfred Bion's concept of 'Container–Contained' (1962; *see* Box 3.2). Bion described the baby's need for 'containment' of overwhelming sense data – pain, hunger, fear, distress – which he does not have the mental apparatus to process or make sense of in any way. He relies on an available, consistent care-giver, usually the parent, who feels the impact of his distress without being overwhelmed by it, who can think about his needs and respond to them. The baby gradually internalises an idea of a thoughtful parental figure who can verbalise his feeling states and modify them in a helpful way. He begins to identify with this figure, becoming eventually more able to perform this function of 'thinking' for himself. Instead of expelling his unbearable feelings through screaming, he may develop a capacity for symbolic thinking, eventually expressing his feelings verbally or through play and drawing.

Feelings of disappointment, shock or depression at news of a damaged baby

> **Box 3.2  The concept of 'Container–Contained' (Bion 1962a)**
>
> The psychoanalyst Wilfred Bion described an unconscious mental process performed automatically by most primary care-givers with their infants. Since a baby has limited mental capacities and can become quickly overwhelmed by a flood of often unpleasant (but also intensely stimulating) sensory experiences, the parent needs to be receptive to these states, think about them and try and make sense of them, returning them to the infant in a more digested, manageable form, by her attentiveness to her baby's fluctuating emotional states. In this way she provides some containment to the infant who internalises, over time, a capacity to reflect on his own states without being overwhelmed by them.

may be difficult for parents to deal with, with the result that instead of providing containment for their infant's unmanageable states, they may unwittingly push out their unprocessed painful feelings into their infant. The infant becomes the receptacle for powerful feelings, which emanate from a care-giver, of disappointment and shock. These, in turn, may impact on the infant and interfere with the bonding relationship between mother and baby. As a result, the baby may take into himself an idea of being a disappointment, unworthy of love, deserving of rejection. In order to protect himself from the invasion of these painful, unprocessed projections, an infant may adopt autistic-type defences, cutting off from contact, or alternatively, may resort to violently expelling uncomfortable or painful feelings by kicking and screaming and later being hyperactive and disruptive – since there is no functioning parental container for his unmanageable feelings. In this way the 'primary handicap' that is the original organic damage is compounded by 'secondary handicap', as the child adopts these defensive strategies to avoid dealing with painful projections and feelings he cannot cope with. This could make these children appear to be more damaged and 'mindless' than they actually are, whilst also masking their true capacities.

## Attacks on thinking

This process of adopting defensive strategies designed to avoid awareness of painful feelings and realities may continue through a child's life, interfering with relationships at home and school. In the classroom, this may manifest in children making unconscious attacks on thinking and on the making of meaningful connections and relationships. Since the main function of a teacher is to encourage the development of meaningful links – and an integrating of ideas – to enhance a student's capacity to think, this can lead to the devaluing of learning and of the teacher's role. The pupils use this attack on thinking to avoid knowing about unbearable truths to do with their own painful predicament, feeling, in many cases, inadequate, incapable and worthless. Thus they adopt their learning 'disability' as a defensive strategy against learning.

## Teacher discussion groups

Discussion groups were offered to the teachers, beginning with the primary school teachers, to help them think about the children in their care. Groups met fortnightly and the teachers, and later support staff, were encouraged to focus on a particular child, recording in detail any observations about or interactions with him during his school day. This included noting the teacher's own emotional responses to the child, which can be valuable indicators of the child's state of mind.

The role of the consultant, using a psychoanalytic model, was to help build up a picture of the child's inner world and an increased understanding of his often unconscious communications. This could, in turn, inform classroom strategy. Apparently incomprehensible behaviour began to make sense, as staff recognised that events and details that may be considered irrelevant or unimportant are often imbued with meaning. Changes of routine, absence of a particular worker, and transitions from home to school or classroom to dining room have an impact on the children.

The teachers were sometimes shocked to notice how easy it was for them to collude with the children's strategies for avoiding mental pain, whereby they would give the impression (again a kind of exaggerated learning disability) that they didn't notice changes of staff, etc., as if it had no meaning for them. It was easier, in some ways, for staff to go along with the children's unconscious attacks on the importance of meaningful relationships because, of course, recognising that children have particular attachment figures, or that it makes a difference who takes the child to the toilet or feeds him, places an extra burden of awareness and thinking on staff. The children use these defence mechanisms to avoid awareness of dependency on important figures to them because this involves tolerating anxiety about the possibility of loss and separation (*see* Box 3.3).

Case study 3.1 provides an example of a discussion meeting, focusing on 13-year-old Chan.

---

**Case study 3.1 Chan, 13 years old**

The classroom staff (one teacher, two assistants) described how Chan, who is one of the more able students, arouses feelings of frustration and despair in them because of his slowness and lack of responsiveness. He turns his back on his fellow pupils, and if addressed by a teacher in class, he slaps his face repeatedly. It is as if he concretely attacks his capacity to think and communicate with others, and resorts to rather autistic types of defences and self-harming behaviour.

The support staff had observed that Chan's favourite activity was to wrap himself in soft sensual fabrics from the dressing-up box, sometimes draping himself in a whole curtain. In contrast to his withdrawn behaviour at other times, he then 'comes to life', dancing and singing in an 'exhibitionistic' way.

---

> **Box 3.3 Defences against thinking and linking (Bion 1962*b*)**
>
> The psychoanalyst Wilfred Bion described how one defence against anxiety (linked to painful awareness of feeling helpless, inadequate and small) may be a process of unconsciously attacking one's own or another's capacity to make meaningful links and connections between ideas and words, or between people in a relationship. This unconscious breaking up of the potential links between people and ideas results in the devaluation of meaningful relationships.

The consultant suggested that Chan may need to feel held tight by the fabrics, as if by another layer of skin, to hold him together before he can 'let go' and express himself. (Perhaps he has an idea of being right 'inside' something or someone, completely merged with them, thus avoiding the painful difficulties of separation.) He immerses himself in a sensation-dominated world, enveloped in silky fabrics and arousing music. This tactile and auditory world of pleasurable sensations takes the place of a relationship with another person, enabling him to evade what could be meaningful but also difficult contact with staff and pupils.

Staff described how Chan would not leave the dining hall after lunch as if stuck to his seat. The consultant suggested that the firm framework of the chair seems to hold him together in the absence of an internal holding structure, just as the structure of the classroom and the routine of lunchtime provide a kind of 'holding' or containment. He may be frightened of outside spaces, an unstructured 'playtime', and may feel as if he could simply fall apart if he unsticks himself from the chair, hence his refusal to go out and play (*see* Box 3.4).

The teacher also described struggling to elicit a response from Chan, despite her certainty that he knew the correct answer, resulting in him eventually chanting the answer in a mocking way. She would calmly praise him, encouraging him to say the word properly, whilst feeling increasingly angry at his pantomime antics. The consultant suggested that his response seemed to make a fool of her and to devalue her work. Chan seemed to be rubbishing the teacher's efforts to help him think, whilst idealising the sensual enveloping fabrics into which he escapes.

The consultant suggested that Chan might respond positively to the teacher showing him that she can tell the difference between when he's genuinely trying to learn and when he's mocking her efforts. In this way she would demonstrate to

> **Box 3.4 Second skin defences (Bick 1967)**
>
> Esther Bick described how in the absence of a containing, thoughtful adult available to help an infant/child process his difficult emotional states, the child develops alternative ways of coping and holding himself together. He may develop what Bick calls a 'second skin defence', finding his own ways of preventing himself from a feeling of falling apart, by precocious muscular development, hyperactivity (kinetically holding himself together), or sticking himself in an adhesive way to a person or object so that he feels the skin-to-skin contact holds him in one piece.

him that she could retain her capacity to think, despite his projections of 'foolishness' into her. The consultant also suggested that Chan would probably pick up the insincerity of her calm 'patient' words, spoken while she was feeling such understandable rage towards him.

It may be more helpful for the teacher to acknowledge her feelings of anger and frustration stirred up through these interactions, and recognise these as useful clues to gauge Chan's state of mind. It is possible that Chan projects his feelings into her in the hope that she will understand and verbalise them. In this way she may then become aware of Chan's feelings of anger, frustration and helplessness and he may feel his emotional states have been understood and contained.

The staff felt relieved by the discussion of the importance of monitoring their own emotional states, as they had felt they were failing professionally by becoming angry and impatient. The consultant described Chan being like a baby who doesn't have the mental capacity to cope with feelings of upset or anger, but gets rid of them by pushing them into others, who are filled with rage while he remains cut off and apparently unperturbed. When an attempt is made to help him think and make connections, he veers away from it. If he begins to think, the truth about his damage might feel more painful than he can tolerate.

The mood in the group shifted as staff then recalled painful moments. For example, staff remembered that when they were giving out Christmas presents, Chan was convinced there wouldn't be one for him. It was wondered if this was his way of defending against disappointment or perhaps it was linked to his unconscious awareness of his attacks on his teacher's capacities, which could bring about retaliation.

Staff related that Chan's mother was reluctant for Chan to go on any school outings because she didn't want him to be seen in public with other disabled children. This seems to be a painful case of a parent being unable to mourn the healthy child that wasn't born and welcome the child who replaced it. Chan must have felt inadequate and a disappointment to his parents and he was powerfully projecting these feelings into the teacher, who then felt undermined by these feelings of inadequacy. She told the consultant guiltily that it sometimes felt easier to give up her efforts and get on with the next child.

When the consultant heard about Chan several months later, the teacher reported many improvements, saying that the staff had been more able to monitor and think about the emotional impact he was having on them and had been trying to use this to understand Chan's own emotional states. This had led, they felt, to more sincere, genuine interchanges with Chan, and an increase in his responsiveness and ability to interact intelligently with the teacher, who felt correspondingly more motivated to persevere with him. They told the consultant that Chan's mother had been amazed by his ability to think and act intelligently on a recent outing with her to a restaurant. Chan had found his way unaided to the toilet to be sick after overeating, missed the toilet bowl and returned to his mother to let her know there was a mess that needed clearing up.

As a result of being thought about and feeling his emotional 'mess' had been contained, Chan was able to demonstrate an increased capacity to think for himself. This may link to the staff themselves feeling that they had a space, with the consultant, to discuss their feelings about this child, which could be used in a constructive way.

## Consultation meetings with senior management staff

---

**Case study 3.1 contd.**

Discussion meetings with the teachers progressed well for two years until an end-of-term review when the teachers resisted reviewing the children's progress and used the time to express their own feelings of disgruntlement: they felt undervalued and confused about their roles. Were they meant to be carers or educators? Physical or medical needs often took priority over curriculum needs, and now that an external inspection was due, how would they be perceived in their professional roles dealing with such damaged children? They lacked the enthusiasm to continue meeting and this raised for the consultant the thought that she, too, was meant to feel undervalued and redundant. At around this time the head teacher requested a consultation after a member of staff had been assaulted by a child in school. It was suggested that a forum for discussing how to support the teachers, who were clearly feeling 'battered', albeit not physically, could be helpful. The teachers were clearly communicating that unless they felt supported and understood they could not attend to the needy children in their care.

---

Four meetings were offered to the management staff of the school (consisting of the head teacher, deputy head and heads of nursery, primary and secondary sections). The aim was to consider the role of management in supporting teachers, who in turn needed to provide support to the classroom assistants and children. A brief summary will be given of these four meetings, highlighting the themes that emerged.

### First meeting

In the first meeting, the consultant heard from a management perspective about the differences in teachers' capacities to deal with exposure to intense levels of mental pain. Some teachers come to the work burdened with personal difficulties; many are gifted with sensitivity and intuition. It emerged that traditionally classroom assistants were responsible for the physical care of the children, toileting, feeding, etc., freeing up the teacher to run curriculum activities. The consultant commented that the assistants may represent the sensual, physical experience of the children, whilst the teachers represented mental life and the value of thinking. The teachers' disgruntlement seemed to be understandable in the light of the very real priorities that physical care sometimes took over teaching, with medication needing to be administered and physiotherapy provided at specific times. In addition, teachers of children with learning disabilities sometimes feel themselves to be 'the bottom of the heap'.

  Through the consultant's questions about the school structure, details about the internal hierarchy between support staff, and some tension between teachers, who could feel undermined as well as supported by support staff, emerged. Support staff, though less qualified, are usually older than the teachers and difficulties around where real authority and power were held became clear. The head teacher described feeling upset to think that teachers 'get far less job satisfaction than they deserve'.

The consultant suggested that parents of handicapped children might feel at times that they too get little satisfaction from their children. She described how in the earliest relationship between a mother and her damaged baby, unbearable feelings of disappointment – too painful to think about – can be projected into the infant. These unbearable feelings can get pushed out, in turn by children into staff, so that staff are given an experience of feeling disappointed and inadequate at their task, as parents often do. Staff may be the receptacles of projections from parents who feel that they too get less satisfaction from their children than they had expected, especially as painful discrepancies in achievement become more evident as children grow older. This was acknowledged with relief by the senior staff group.

## Second meeting

The second meeting began with a discussion about levels of teacher competence. The consultant suggested that teachers could be feeling undermined by their assistants, who may believe that what they do is more important than what the teachers do. She suggested that this overvaluing of one kind of approach (physical care, instant gratification) and undervaluing of another (mental creativity and making meaningful connections) might originate from a more disturbed side of the children themselves. In this state of mind the children may unconsciously launch attacks on the value of thinking. Children may behave in ways that make staff feel it doesn't matter who takes them to the toilet, or sits with them in the dining room, attacking their capacity to think about relatedness and meaningful links. This is because being able to make connections and think could put them in touch with their own unbearable predicament (*see* Box 3.5). Teachers may at times be overwhelmed by projections of inadequacy from the children, which leave them feeling deskilled and inadequate. These feelings of worthlessness may interfere with their true capacities and can be reflected in the quality of their work but may not reflect the teacher's true level of competence.

The head teacher rejected this idea, reiterating that teachers were valued but performance was variable. The consultant stuck to her line of argument, suggesting that anyone who offers a new idea, encouraging thought, like a teacher, is often met initially with hostility. Similarly, this could include the management group in this meeting, resisting her new ideas. At this mention of their own possible resistance to the consultant's ideas, the head teacher suddenly recalled that she had recently herself done a piece of work with a class, which could support them.

---

**Case study 3.1 contd.**

The head teacher had begun to do some work on a children's story, 'Peter and the Wolf', set to music (Prokofiev), a simple narrative with different relationships between characters. All went well initially, but in the final phase, as the piece was gelling into a cohesive whole, the children's behaviour became disruptive. The head decided that she had made an error of judgement, the work was beyond the children's limited capacities and she should perhaps have stuck to a simpler task. However, on discussing her misgivings with other teachers, they persuaded her to persevere, saying the work was proving to be successful and they had noticed the children's development through the experience. With their support she completed the project well.

From this example it was possible to recognise how easy it is to underestimate the capacities of damaged children, by mistaking their unconscious attacks on thinking for actual organic damage – congenital 'stupidity'. The escalation of disruptive attacks, just when the linking narrative was beginning to cohere, may reflect the children's attempts to avoid awareness of painful truths to do with damage and loss. As the story involved the characters using physical agility and a lively intelligence to escape a fierce wolf, the children's own limitations in such a situation could be highlighted. This kind of attack can result in children depriving themselves of further opportunities for development, unless teachers are supported in noticing and understanding the meaning of their behaviour, and are encouraged to persevere with activities promoting thinking. The staff group could also note how easy it is to underestimate a teacher's capacities when he/she is under the sway of such powerful projections.

The management team then wondered about those teachers who, unlike the head teacher who had sought help, may succumb to countless attacks on their

---

**Box 3.5 Defences against thinking**

Babies and young children who do not have enough experiences of a consistent care-giver who provides attentive containment of their over-whelming states may develop defensive strategies to deal with this 'primary disappointment'. A baby may resort to challenging disruptive or hyperactive behaviour as he attempts to force his feelings into an unreceptive carer, with increasing intensity. He may become withdrawn and cut himself off from 'knowing about' painful feelings of disappointment or loss by cutting off from meaningful contact with others. This makes the task of a teacher, in engaging a child with the process of making meaningful connections, particularly difficult.

These attacks on thinking can take the form of unconscious projections into teachers of feelings of incompetence and inadequacy. Teachers can feel that their task, which is to promote thinking and make connections, is devalued and can be filled with projections of inadequacy. These feelings of inadequacy and failure can be profoundly undermining if staff are not helped to recognise them as projections from children, rather than reflections of their inherent competence. This process can lead to an overvaluing of mindless sensory experience, as opposed to thinking and making creative connections, and can filter up from the children, through classroom assistants and teachers, and into the management structure of the institution, permeating every level of functioning at the school.

work without being consciously aware of them happening. It was concluded that there may be some teachers who feel confident in their creativity and can withstand the attacks, managing to contain and process some of the projections they receive with the occasional input from the consultant and the educational therapist. However, there may be those who are perfectly competent but who feel insecure and thus are prone to take projections of inadequacy personally. The role of team leaders as an essential support to the teachers became clear.

### Third meeting

The discussions progressed to consider the nature of the support that teachers may need from their team leaders. How could teachers be helped to be aware of the unconscious resistance in pupils to thinking and linking, without feeling overwhelmed by their task? How could they be aware of the powerful projections into them from pupils (often an accurate gauge of the child's emotional state) without feeling overburdened by insight?

The consultant suggested that although it is necessary to accept the fact of primary organic damage, there is a way of helping children give up their 'secondary handicaps' (Sinason 1992) and move towards emotional truth and understanding. Individual child psychotherapy with a child referred from the school was described. Once this child's well-established autistic defences against pain began to break down, she became more in touch with feelings of loss and separation and became increasingly vulnerable as a result.

This theme was then broadened to an institutional level, drawing a parallel with the risks to vulnerable staff, who may open themselves up to experiencing the painful projections of the children and may feel overwhelmed as a result. Just as children have a need of their defences to protect them from unbearable pain, the same could be true of staff. The management team agreed that there is a similar risk for staff members, who may not be able to cope with the increasing levels of mental pain they receive once they are helped to be more receptive to the children's communications, and may cut themselves off from the emotional needs of their pupils perhaps as a defence against too much pain and disturbance.

It was suggested that those who remain defensively cut off may unwittingly provoke disruptive behaviour as children intensify their efforts to be understood by violently forcing their feelings into an apparently unresponsive teacher. It was agreed that ongoing support from the senior staff team was essential if one was going to encourage this kind of increased emotional awareness in staff.

The consultations were able to explore a tightening of the management structure to help provide a safe, boundaried setting within which to provide containment for the powerful projections from children, staff and parents. This implies acknowledging a 'vertical' hierarchical structure, moving away from an illusion of a 'horizontal' structure where an impression is given that everyone has equal status. As sometimes happens in schools for children with special needs, there is an effort made to offer a kind of homely intimacy in the school, which can lead to a blurring of boundaries, giving confusing messages about hierarchy and authority figures (horizontal structure). Staff, including the head teacher, are all addressed by their first names, and some parents of pupils are employed in the school in a range of capacities. Classroom assistants often double as foster parents or respite carers for some pupils and many teachers have entered this profession because of personal experiences with learning disabled children, often in their own families.

The head described parents coming into the office without appointments, often anxious or angry, and her feeling that she has to attend to them immediately, that they cannot wait. Setting firm boundaries – saying 'no' – was acknowledged as a problem, reflecting the serious difficulties many parents were experiencing in this area, where their children had become tyrannical, greedy, intrusive and out of control. An integrated approach with a firm, non-punitive line of authority (with the head and deputy head assuming, in the metaphor of family relationships, a parental rather than a sibling role) was recognised as more helpful. The management group acknowledged that in order to provide containment within the school, they too need to feel contained within a supportive firm structure, which could include ongoing input from the consultant.

The teachers' reluctance to continue their discussion meetings with the consultant was explored as a similar resistance to new perspectives that might be offered. If one didn't take the rejection personally, it could be seen as a communication of the teachers' experience in the classroom with pupils who devalue the teachers' new ideas. The head said she didn't think the teachers were resisting seeing the consultant, but that they were feeling depressed and deflated. It was possible to discuss how the teachers were communicating a wish for support which did not involve anything too painful or penetrative like a new idea – this would be felt as hard and cruel – but rather a wish for comfort and sympathy, the 'receptive' aspect of containment.

This led to a discussion of how easily a split can occur between the deputy head and the head; where the latter can be perceived as tough and demanding, the former is approached for support and comfort. The consultant commented on the contrast between the head teacher's perceived role of being the 'head', the thinking mind, in contrast to the deputy head, who is perceived as offering instant gratification and sensory comfort to the teachers. This encouraged further ways of thinking about support for staff from year heads, and support for year heads from the head teacher and deputy head teacher, who jointly provide the leadership within the school.

## Fourth meeting

An example of the pull towards sensory comfort, and away from more demanding mental activity, emerged at the highest level of management in our fourth and final meeting. The head, chatting to the consultant informally before the meeting began, commented on how 'nice and comforting' it was to be doing the deputy head's duties (who was ill). These involve going around and distributing supplies of wipes, cleaning materials, disinfectants, etc. 'You get such instant satisfaction!' she exclaimed. When the two roles were considered, it was noted that they are divided so that the deputy head looks after the internal running of the school, including practical aspects, whilst the head is responsible for external liaison. It was possible to see how the head needed to always hold in mind a dual vision – of the 'normal' world of education and development, as well as the values and needs of the particular pupils in her school, and how this could, at times, be distressing.

In considering future plans, everyone recognised that poor staff relationships could have an impact on the effective implementation of any curriculum changes, and that the particular emotional disturbances of the pupils meant that staff support was important.

## Outcome of management meetings

The impact on the teacher group was noticeable as they became increasingly confident and empowered. Over the past two years the role of the team leaders has been refined. At the same time, the management structure has become tighter and more defined, resulting in many positive developments as well as a whole new raft of problems, which is the inevitable result of a clarifying of differences within the management structure. However, the impact of closer communication between the head, deputy head teacher and senior staff members (besides information-giving briefs) has ensured that new ideas are discussed, thought about and contained within the senior staff group before they are introduced to teachers, support staff and, finally, to the children.

The school head acknowledged the benefits of using a therapeutic model in the way it has been developed in her school. She stressed that the process of integrating the therapeutic input with policy making and practice in order to arrive at a workable model was a long and difficult one, but well worthwhile. She felt the work enabled the management team to consider the effect on the staff group of exposure to the physically and emotionally challenging behaviours of some children and the ways in which they transferred their distress onto staff members. This then enabled the management team to look carefully at situations where staff were under particular pressure and to offer additional support, and opportunities to think and talk.

---

### Learning points

- Primitive unconscious processes and defence mechanisms resorted to in early infancy, possibly as a result of difficulties in the early mother–infant relationship, can impact on the functioning of teaching and management staff and on the institution as a whole.
- This may result in teachers feeling undervalued and deskilled. It may be a reflection of the children's need to defend themselves against awareness of painful realities by unconsciously attacking those who promote thinking activities. It may not be a reflection of teachers' real capacities.
- An understanding of this dynamic may enable teachers to avoid taking personally these attacks on their professional capacities and to understand them as communications from the children about their worries and ways of coping with unmanageable anxieties.
- It can give teachers additional tools for understanding children's behaviour.
- It can increase teachers' confidence in their own observational abilities and endorse their emotional experience of a child in the classroom as valid.
- Since teachers have more frequent contact with their pupils than an outside professional, an enhanced understanding of their pupils'

emotional needs can be greatly beneficial. The teacher is able to provide more 'containment' for the children in his/her classroom.

- It is helpful to have a framework for thinking that enables these dynamics to be recognised and reflected on by professionals working with these troubled and needy children.

## Consultation to a school for academic excellence

The consultant's role in this school focused on helping the staff to think about children they were concerned about, and seeing the children for individual 'counselling'. The consultation meetings with teachers usually followed a referral of a pupil by the headmaster (in discussion with the relevant teacher and year head), and served the dual purpose of enabling the consultant and consultee to think together about their concerns, as well as providing the consultant with information about the child's areas of difficulty at school.

There was considerable emphasis placed on the children's academic performance and in meetings with teachers (and parents and children) the discrepancy between many of the children's academic abilities and their emotional needs was noticeable. Some pupils used their intellectual capacities to conceal their feelings of vulnerability from others (and from themselves) and to create the impression of being in control, particularly when circumstances in their home lives meant that things were largely out of their control. It soon became clear that discussion meetings to help teachers think about the children in their class were not going to feature in this highly academic, pressurised environment, which could not allow for the timetabling of this kind of input.

When taking on a referral, the consultant always met briefly with the class teacher, and, where possible, encouraged him/her to attend the meeting with the parents and to contribute their observations of the child. After completing her assessment, she would feed back to parents and meet briefly with the teacher and school nurse, who seemed to represent the pastoral voice of the school. As time went on, the consultant tried to involve staff in fuller discussions as a group. She also began to use classroom observation, in those classes where it would not be felt as a threat to the teacher, as a method of understanding some of the children's difficulties, as well as a way of involving the teachers in the process.

The case study that follows illustrates how an initial consultation meeting with staff concerned about a child provided some 'containment' (Bion 1962a) for the class teacher, and offered a framework for thinking about the child's situation both at school and at home. This then led to a meeting with the parents and some direct work with the child.

Case study 3.2  Peter

In a school where the focus was on the children's academic skills, the role of the consultant as someone concerned with emotional matters was often marginalised until a crisis occurred, when there would be an urgent request to try and resolve a situation. Such a situation occurred with Peter, a bright

*Continued*

eight-year-old who had suddenly become very disruptive in his music classes. This had culminated in him throwing a musical instrument at his teacher during a music lesson, narrowly missing her eye.

## Staff consultation meeting

The consultant had an initial meeting with the year head and teacher to gain some background to this event. She heard that Peter had been difficult with this teacher especially since returning to school from a recent holiday break.

Through careful questioning, it became clear that Peter saw this teacher more often than most other teachers (in this school classes had a different teacher for each subject). The consultant suggested the possibility that he may have formed a particular attachment to her, as a maternal figure in a male-dominated school, resulting in him feeling let down and angry when he didn't see her over the long holiday period. Children can often feel abandoned, by teachers to whom they have formed an attachment, over the holiday period. The teacher agreed, saying that, interestingly, when he was in trouble with her, he had whispered sadly: ' I let you down'. The consultant suggested that feeling let down, and then letting others down, seemed to be an important communication in his behaviour. The year head described Peter standing on the stairs, blocking other boys' path up to the classroom. The teacher talked about a new baby brother at home, describing how when Peter's father came to collect him after school, carrying the infant in his arms, he trailed far behind his father, as if he wasn't all connected with the father and did not feel held in his mind.

The consultant suggested that Peter might be transferring onto the teacher and the classroom situation his fears about being displaced and neglected at home, because of the new baby. Having to share a teacher with 20 other children can be difficult for young children at the best of times, but during this sensitive period Peter may have felt that he had to gain and hold his teacher's attention at all costs.

Just as Peter seems to feel his father can only hold one child in mind at any one time, and so cannot attend to him when he has the new baby in his arms, so he might feel that his teacher cannot pay attention to all the children in her care. If she's attending to another child or not paying direct attention to him, he might imagine that he has been completely forgotten. Therefore a kind of possessive jealousy and determination to keep himself in the front of her mind always, by whichever means, takes over. His throwing the musical instrument and his blocking off of others from access to the teacher may be his way of communicating his need to keep all his rival pupils at bay by whatever means. They also convey feelings of jealousy and fears about emotional neglect that threaten to overwhelm him. In his current state of mind, he does not have the capacity to think about or verbalise his feelings – on the contrary, he gets rid of them out of himself into others. The teacher is meant to have an experience of being hurt and shocked perhaps so that she can understand what it feels like for Peter, who is alerting her to the fact that he is experiencing an emotional crisis.

It seemed important that Peter was not allowed to take up all of the teacher's time and attention, since she needed to demonstrate that, in fact, she was able to keep all the children, including Peter, in mind.

The teacher found some of these ideas helpful, as she felt that she could understand some of the underlying emotional basis for the sudden deterioration in Peter's behaviour. She could not condone this behaviour or allow him to monopolise her attention in the classroom or cause injury or damage. However, understanding that much of his disruptive behaviour was a result of his possibly unconscious need to get rid of his rivals for her attention could alter her strategies in the classroom. For example, she might consider how putting him out of the class at the first sign of disruption would simply be an enactment of the feelings of exclusion and rejection that he hopes she will 'receive' from him and understand. Placing him in the very front of the class, with a clear view of her, and where she can quickly apprehend the early signs of disruption before they escalate, could be helpful. The teacher seemed to feel that her own distress had been contained to some extent.

Bearing these thoughts in mind, the consultant met with Peter's parents, who emphasised their close relationship with him and acknowledged how the birth of baby Jason may have affected him badly. They agreed to an individual assessment of Peter's emotional needs, followed by a feedback meeting. An extract from the first meeting with Peter illustrates how consultation can usefully inform individual work and vice versa.

## Individual assessment meetings with Peter

He is a small boy with a bright open face and he came in laden with a huge book on 'The Battle of Britain' and began to draw the British flag.

---

**Case study 3.2 contd.**

The consultant suggested that he had introduced the idea of battles with this book and perhaps battles at school or at home might be in his mind.

He agreed, saying that he got annoyed at home because he had to help mum change the baby's dirty nappies.

The consultant addressed his feelings of annoyance at the new baby's arrival.

Peter complained that his crying at night kept him awake which is why he wished to move bedrooms. He drew a plan of his house, indicating where his current bedroom was and where he was hoping to move to, speaking in quite an adult way.

The consultant pointed out that in fact Peter was saying he wanted to move to a room closer to his parents' room, where mum, dad and baby Jason were all sleeping.

He quickly interjected, saying 'it's a bigger room, with better heating'.

The consultant suggested that perhaps his difficulty sleeping at night was linked to a feeling of being 'left out in the cold': he can't sleep without the nice, warm, cosy feelings of being near to mum and dad.

He nodded sadly.

The consultant suggested that feeling left out seemed to him the same as being forgotten about, and this gave him a cold, 'pushed-out' feeling.

He nodded.

---

*Continued*

The consultant suggested that he may feel the same way in his teacher's class, causing him to move in close to her to make sure he didn't get left out, just like he wanted to move bedroom to be closer to his parents.

He agreed, talking quietly and saying that when he was in his room he overheard his parents saying nasty things about him. The consultant wondered whether something similar happened at school: when he was feeling bad he might imagine others were saying horrible things about him and that could lead to battles at school.

He agreed.

She suggested that things had been very difficult for Peter at school.

He then told her that although it appeared as if he was angry, in reality he was feeling upset.

'So, when you throw things it's to make sure someone else is upset and hurt so they can understand how you're feeling?' (Peter nodded.)

The consultant suggested he might also wonder whether she would like him and want to see him again, assuring him about their next appointment.

He said he wanted to do a very special drawing and that was why he had taken the book out of the library.

The consultant asked if he felt his teacher would then think he was a very special boy, the best in the class, and he agreed.

She suggested that was how he may have felt at home before Jason had been born, his parents' special baby, and then suddenly mum and dad had made another one.

He smiled and nodded.

The consultant said perhaps he needed to think he was special and he could do that with his drawing.

He suddenly looked around and noticed other drawings pinned around the room.

The consultant pointed out that suddenly he had become aware that, instead of being in a room together just the two of them, he was aware of being surrounded by other children's art, as if they were all in competition for her attention. As if in response, he told her that he wondered what the rest of the class was doing, and soon the meeting time was over.

In following meetings, Peter's anger towards his baby brother emerged more clearly in the material. He drew pictures of air force battles where the small ('baby') plane would be isolated from the couple of larger (parent) planes and middle-sized (brother) plane, and, caught out by a bright spotlight, it would be shot down in flames. The consultant was able to take up Peter's concerns about the baby being in the spotlight at home, and his angry feelings towards his young sibling. The consultant addressed with Peter how strongly he felt about there not being enough space in mummy's mind for both Peter and his brother – he had to get rid of his rival.

After four of these individual meetings with Peter the consultant met with his parents and the year head to give feedback. They expressed gratitude that the school and the consultant had alerted them to the fact that Peter was going through a crisis, and acknowledged how much things had improved at school and at home. Peter had been able to express his feelings of rage and jealousy through his drawings, thereby reducing the amount of acting out in the classroom. The teacher was able to see that throwing Peter out of the classroom confirmed his worst fears, and that she was acting on his projections of rejection – rejecting him, when what he needed most was to be kept close and well in focus by her.

---

**Learning points**

- Consultation to staff in organisations can help them to understand the meaning of children's play and behaviour.
- Sometimes the consultation work provides sufficient input for staff who are then enabled to provide the necessary support to children and their families as well as other staff members. No further therapeutic intervention may be required.
- This has the benefit of empowering staff and increasing their skill base as they gain new perspectives and insights into children's psychological states. Teachers develop the resources to tackle some problems themselves without involving outside professionals.
- In some situations consultation may highlight a need for further work. However, the initial consultation work with senior managers and staff members is an essential preliminary to further work because it establishes between the professionals a joint basis for understanding the area of the child's difficulties.
- If further work is required, it is important to ensure that the work of the consultant has the full support of parents, teachers and senior management staff if it is going to be effective. It is therefore essential that a strong alliance is first established between the consultant, and the staff/management of a school. The initial consultation meeting usually creates this solid foundation, resulting in a joint understanding of the problems and an endorsement by senior managers of the fact that further therapeutic work (however brief) is required.

---

## Conclusion: the use of observational skills

In the introduction to this chapter mention was made of how the psycho-analytic tools used for understanding individuals in a psychotherapeutic context can be applied to an understanding of institutional dynamics. One of the central tools in this work is the development of acutely honed observational skills. As a prerequisite to all child and many adult psychotherapy trainings in Britain, students are required to undertake an infant observation, observing an infant in his/her home for an hour once-weekly for up to two years. The attention to minute detail in the baby's behaviour and to the developing interaction between parent and baby is later transferred to clinical situations, where clinicians are required to be receptive to a range of intense emotional states in their clients.

These skills can also be transferred to consultation settings. The consultant attempts to elicit detailed observations from staff during a consultation meeting (see, for example, Case study 3.1). Staff are often surprised at how much detailed observational material they can produce. The group discussion provides an opportunity to think about the meaning of what they have observed and to try to think about what the child is communicating about his emotional experience. Staff often gain enough insight to be able to continue the work without further therapeutic input being required for the children. If further therapeutic input is required, the initial consultation provides a solid basis for a supportive framework to be created around the child and professional engaged in the therapeutic work.

As we saw in the first section, at times consultation at the highest managerial level is required in order to effect changes in the structure of the organisation. These changes are usually in the interest of providing clear boundaries and greater emotional containment for staff, and thereby, to the pupils in their care.

In the second example, by contrast, we saw how a very particular personal internal drama within one child was being enacted in a destructive way within the school. Once an understanding was gained of the meaning of his behaviour, strategies could be put in place which altered the classroom dynamics and supported the teacher in her role.

Although the examples given arise from very different schools, with a different pupil population and different goals, consultation offered a valuable opportunity for staff of each school to reflect on the dynamics operating within the school, as well as within individual children.

## References

Bick E (1967) The experiences of the skin in early object relations. In: *Collected Papers of Martha Harris and Esther Bick*. Roland Harris Education Trust, London.

Bion WR (1962*a*) *Learning from Experience*. Heinemann, London. Reprinted: Karnac, London, 1984.

Bion WR (1962*b*) A theory of thinking. *International Journal of Psychoanalysis*. 43: 306–10. In: *Second Thoughts*. Karnac, London, 1964. Also in: *Melanie Klein Today, Vol. 1*. Routledge, London, 1988.

Sinason V (1992) *Mental Handicap and the Human Condition: new approaches from the Tavistock*. Free Association Books, London.

# Chapter 4

# Consultation: a solution-focused approach

*Evan George*

## Introduction

The birth of solution-focused brief therapy was announced to the world in the pages of the Journal *Family Process* in 1986 (de Shazer *et al.* 1986). The approach has a clear and distinguished family history including, amongst its forebears, Milton Erikson, the American hypnotherapist, and Gregory Bateson, the English anthropologist along with his many celebrated colleagues in the Schizophrenic Communication Project, most notably John Weakland and Paul Watzlawick. It was Weakland and Watzlawick who founded the Mental Research Institute at Palo Alto and who developed their own brief therapy, a problem-resolution approach (Weakland *et al.* 1974) that was the clearest pregenitor of solution-focused brief therapy. And yet it is to Steve de Shazer and Insoo Kim Berg, from the Milwaukee Brief Family Therapy Center, that the greatest acknowledgement must be given for bringing the approach into being. Since 1986 the influence of solution-focused brief therapy has grown rapidly across the world as its flexibility, effectiveness and consumer and user-friendliness have been recognised. Whilst initially viewed as a family therapy, clinicians quickly realised that the approach could also be used with individuals, couples and indeed in groups. The flexibility of the approach has become increasingly apparent as leaders in the field have described its application in an ever-widening range of areas: education (Rhodes and Ajmal 1995; Ajmal and Rees 2001), neglect and abuse (Turnell and Edwards 1999), eating difficulties (Jacob 2001), family breakdown (Berg 1994), problem drinking and drug use (Berg and Miller 1992; Berg and Reuss 1997). Latterly it has become apparent that solution-focused brief therapy is more than merely a collection of techniques, that contained within it there is a way of thinking and that this way of thinking can be applied to a wide range of 'non-therapy' situations, most notably consultation, supervision, team-building, coaching and indeed to many management processes. This development has been marked by the appearance of the first solution-focused text dealing with the wider world of business and business consulting (McKergow and Jackson 2002).

This chapter deals with the application of solution-focused thinking to the process of consultation and will start with an overview of the approach. It will then consider how the solution-focused approach is put to work in consultation before going on to explore an example of consultation to the senior management team of a secondary school.

## Solution-focused brief therapy

Solution-focused brief therapy has been described in a number of ways. Some authors have tended to describe it substantially in terms of a set of techniques (Walter and Peller 1992) while Lipchik (1994), for example, has attempted to describe the approach in terms of a characteristic collection of underlying assumptions. Whilst both of these ways of describing the approach have their strengths, clarity and flexibility seem to be best served by describing the approach as a conversational process. This process is best characterised as one within which the worker attempts to engage the consultee, who typically arrives *problem-dominated*, in a number of very specific forms of solution-focused talking. The shift involved can be described as moving out of problem-talk into solution-talk (*see* Box 4.1).

---

**Box 4.1 Problem domination to solution orientation**

When faced with a problem that we are unable to resolve, it seems not unusual for us to focus increasingly on the problem over a period of time, examining and exploring it, turning it this way and that. We become so familiar with its parameters that when we recognise small parts of the problem pattern we say to ourselves 'here we go again'. Repetition becomes a central part of our experience. This process is often accompanied by increasing engagement in 'problem-talk', discussing the problem, its effects, its patterning and its inevitability. The more that we do this, the larger the problem can appear to be and the more helpless and hopeless we can feel ourselves to be in the face of it.

Solution orientation is achieved through an exploration of preferred futures, a focusing on actions that we are already taking that are useful, a highlighting of progress. Solution orientation is active whilst problem domination tends to be passive. Solution-talk focuses on the future, on useful actions, and seeks to build an expectation of good outcome.

---

Within solution-focused brief therapy, it is suggested that maximising the amount of solution-talk in therapy conversations is associated with a better chance of good outcome (Lipchik 1988). The shift from problem domination to solution orientation is organised around four key themes (*see* Box 4.2).

These four conversational pathways support the shift from problem-talk to solution-talk and form the foundation of the solution-focused process. It should be added that the solution-focused worker will characteristically, in addition, give constructive feedback to the consultee at the end of the session, highlighting in the feedback any evidence gleaned from the session which supports an expectation of progress in the consultee's preferred direction. Finally, it should be stressed that it is not the view of the solution-focused worker that they are solving the consultee's problem. Rather, it is characteristically assumed that if the worker can engage the consultee in solution-talk, the consultee thereby has an enhanced chance of resolving their own problem. The worker engages the consultee in the talk and then lets them get on with the change. The application to the process of consultation is substantially straightforward.

Box 4.2  Key conversational themes

- The first theme involves shifting out of the world of deficit towards a constant interest in and exploration of the resources that the consultee brings to the therapeutic process. It is assumed that the consultee can only ever achieve change by drawing on their resources. Resources are therefore invariably central to the change process and so the solution-focused worker is consistently engaged in a process whereby the consultee is invited to be noticing of and naming of those resources.
- Crucially the consultee is also invited through the questioning to move away from a focus on complaint to a focus on preferred future, detailing the future that they desire rather than the problem past, away from which they typically wish to move.
- Rather than following the consultee in exploring those 'wrong' actions that might be causing or maintaining the problem, the worker's questions invite the consultee to begin to notice anything which is being done that is useful in moving in the direction of their preferred future and which they could therefore usefully do more of.
- Solution-focused brief therapy also takes the view that highlighting progress in therapy is more associated with further change than focusing on 'stuckness'. The approach therefore makes extensive use of specific questions which serve to highlight even the smallest changes in the direction of the preferred future.

## Solution-focused thinking in consultation

### Constructing a context of collaboration

Solution-focused thinking is entirely non-normative. It has within it no way of conceptualising problems; problems are viewed simply as things that people want to change. Since the solution-focused worker can have no view as to what the consultee should want, the worker will always have to ask, and it is not until the consultee has responded that the worker can know in what direction to focus their questioning. The worker must, in this way, be commissioned by the consultee.

The collaborative context extends much further, however, than simply asking the consultee what is wanted. The consultant will typically also take feedback during the process and at the end of the meeting, checking that the consultation is on track and focusing in the right areas. The consultant might similarly enquire of the consultee's experience of previous consultation, seeking to establish what has been found useful in the past and what has not (*see* Box 4.3). Such feedback is subsequently drawn upon as guidance.

### Detailing the preferred future

Having established what the consultee wants from the consultative process, the solution-focused consultant seeks to invite a detailed picture of how it would

> **Box 4.3 Questions**
>
> - What are your best hopes for this meeting?
> - How will you know that this consultation has been useful?
> - What difference are you hoping that our discussion will make to your work with this (client)?
> - Are we talking about the right things?
> - What, if anything, in our meeting today had been of any use to you?
> - In previous consultations what have you found useful?

become clear that the commission had been successfully achieved. For instance, if the consultee were to have stated that their 'best hopes' were that they would be making progress in a 'stuck' piece of work, the solution-focused consultant would seek to establish a detailed picture of how such progress would show itself.

Routinely, in order to enrich the picture of the preferred future, the consultee is invited to describe progress from a range of perspectives, typically including themselves, the client, their manager or supervisor, and other key persons in the client's life.

Enriching the picture of the preferred outcome by developing a description that becomes more and more detailed opens up a constantly widening range of options for action. It also seems that signs of progress, once specified, are more likely to be noticed and thus the consultee can begin to be curious as to what is being done that is working in the situation (*see* Box 4.4).

> **Box 4.4 Questions**
>
> - So how will you know that you are making progress?
> - What signs of progress might you hope to see?
> - What else will tell you that you are making progress?
> - What will the client be doing differently that will tell you that progress is being made?
> - How will you respond differently to the client when you are making progress?
> - How will the client know that you are noticing progress?
> - Who else will notice the progress?
> - What will they see?
> - What will be the first tiny signs that you are making progress in this piece of work?
> - What other tiny signs might there be?
> - How do you imagine that your client will know that things are going well for them?
> - How do you imagine that the client's parents (or teachers or friends) might know?

## What's working

Having established what the consultee wants from the consultation and having developed a picture of this preferred outcome, the solution-focused consultant will seek to invite the consultee to determine what small parts of the successful outcome are already in place or occur sometimes. It might be appropriate to enquire, for instance, 'What signs of progress have you already noticed?' And having established the presence of some signs of progress – however tiny – that the consultee has already noticed, the consultant will begin to enquire, 'What were you doing that might in some way be associated with the progress already made?'

Beginning to establish what the consultee might already have done that is useful helps to establish what the consultee might usefully do more of (*see* Box 4.5).

---

**Box 4.5 Questions**

- What progress have you already noticed?
- In what ways has the situation improved, even a little?
- When are the times that you are feeling more hopeful?
- What are you noticing at these times of 'more hopefulness'?
- What do you think that you might have done that has supported the progress made?
- If I were to ask your client, what do you think that they would say that you have done that has been helpful in some way?

---

## When nothing seems to be working

On some occasions the consultee might not be able to identify anything that they are doing that is useful. Perhaps there has been no progress in the piece of work or things have not gone according to plan. In this case, the solution-focused consultant might choose to widen the focus and begin to invite consideration of what has been done in similar situations in the past that turned out to be useful, or even what the consultee has heard colleagues doing in similar situations that has proved useful.

Attempting to establish what the consultee is already doing that 'is working' might lead to an exploration of what they have been doing to help prevent deterioration or even, in very tough situations, what they have been doing to help themselves to keep going while searching for a way of moving forward (*see* Box 4.6).

The solution-focused consultant assumes that establishing what the consultee is already doing, or has done, that is useful opens the possibility that the consultee could do more of it. This is likely to be a more economical route to change than attempting to change the consultee's approach to their problem. When we as consultants attempt to offer, or to impose, our own ideas of solution, there is always the danger that our solution might not fit with the consultee's own world view and therefore be unhelpful. Focusing on the useful strategies that the

---

**Box 4.6 Questions**

- What have you been doing that has been stopping things getting worse (or even worse/or even worse than they have got)?
- When you have faced similar dilemmas in the past, what have you done that has been useful?
- When in the past you have found yourself feeling stuck, what has helped you to keep going?
- What ideas have you already had of interventions you have thought of but not tried?
- When colleagues have faced similarly tough situations, what do you recall them having found useful?

---

consultee already has will also serve to support their own sense of their own competence rather than highlighting the skills of the consultant. In Michael White's terms (White 2000), the solution-focused consultant attempts to work from a 'decentralised' position, focusing the consultative conversation on the views, perceptions and strategies of the consultee themselves.

## Scaling progress

The solution-focused consultant typically makes liberal use of *scale questions* to establish progress already achieved, to allow for the exploration of what the consultee has done that is useful and to establish detailed pictures of the way forward. The scale question is the solution-focused consultant's single most useful tool, as confirmed by the consistent feedback both of therapeutic clients and professional consultees. Typically the question is structured in a simple and straightforward way which will most often seek to take account of the consultee's 'best hopes' for the consultation:

> 'On a scale of 0 to 10 with 10 standing for things going as well as you could hope and 0 standing for things going as badly as you could imagine, where do you see things between 0 and 10 at present?'

Interestingly very few clients, and similarly few consultees, respond with the answer that they see things at 0. This immediately opens the way to asking, 'What tells you that things are at 3 on the scale and *not* at 0?' The answer will necessarily focus on signs of possibility and progress and invite questions about what the consultee is doing that is useful. Beyond this, the solution-focused consultant will typically focus on 'How will you know that things have moved just one point nearer 10 on your scale?', thereby inviting the consultee to establish what will be for them the first tiny signs that the situation is moving forward.

Scaling questions are enormously flexible and can be *topped* and *tailed* in an infinitely various way (*see* Box 4.7). For example, it might be useful to ask the consultee, 'If 0 stands for the time that you took this case on and 10 stands for confident closure, where do you see things now between 0 and 10?' or 'If 0 stands for the time that you were most concerned about this piece of work and 10 stands for the piece of work being on track, where do you see things now?' In each case

> **Box 4.7  Scale questions**
>
> Whatever is being scaled, these questions tend to be constructed along the same lines. 0 is construed as the worst, the point that the client or consultee wants to move away from, and 10 is construed as the reality that the consultee wants to achieve. If the answer to the question 'where are you now on that scale' is not 'zero', and it rarely is, then this inevitably means that there has been progress or that the consultee is aware that progress is possible. Enquiring about the respondent's evidence for this statement will always highlight 'what's working'. The consultant can then focus on progress, perhaps picking out the +1 point and the 'good enough' point, inviting the respondent to detail how s/he will know that these points have been reached.

the follow-up questions will be the same: 'What tells you that things are there and not at 0?' (if they are not) and then, 'How will you know that things have moved one point up?'

Asking about confidence in good outcome focuses the consultative conversation on the evidence that the consultee has that the client might change. This tends to highlight changes that the client has already made and resources that the client brings to the work. The question can be made more specific, since having asked, 'On a scale of 0 to 10 with 10 representing you having every confidence in a good outcome for this piece of work and 0 representing your absolute knowledge that no progress is possible, where do you see things now?' If we imagine that the consultee responds with a '4', the solution-focused consultant can then ask first, 'What is it that you know about the client that allows you to have "4" confidence?' and then, 'What is it that you know about yourself that allows you to have "4" confidence in good outcome?'

### Separating process from outcome

In tough situations where good outcome cannot be expected it is often useful to separate case outcome and the worker's input. For example, it can be asked:

> 'On a scale of 0 to 10, with 10 standing for you being confident that you have done everything possible and 0 standing for your certainty that you have done yourself and your client no sort of justice in this piece of work, where would you see things at present?'

Focusing on the consultee's input separate from outcome can allow the consultee to notice that there is little more that they can do, while on other occasions focusing them on what else they could do to be more certain of having 'given of their best'.

## Feeding back

The solution-focused consultant will give the consultee feedback on what they have heard which represents evidence of the possibility of good outcome. This will include what has been learned about the resources of both the consultee and the client as well as what both the consultee and the client are doing that is useful in the situation.

If the consultation is to be ongoing then it may be that the consultant will suggest that the consultee watch out, generically perhaps, for evidence of progress and to notice what they and the client are doing at these moments of perceived progress.

## Simple but not easy

Generally it is recognised that the solution-focused process is *simple*. It entails developing a conversation that moves out of problem domination into solution orientation, highlighting the desired direction for progress and searching for evidence of what is already being done that is useful. However, it is equally generally recognised that the process is not *easy*, demanding from the therapist/consultant advanced conversational skills (*see* Box 4.8).

---

**Box 4.8 Solution-focused conversation**

- The consultant must develop a repertoire of specifically solution-oriented questions.
- The consultant must constantly frame questions that are simultaneously sufficiently close to the consultee's world-view to make sense to the consultee and sufficiently distinct in order for the possibility of difference to occur.
- The consultant must resist any urge to be more expert than the consultee, restricting themselves to asking useful questions, the answering of which on the part of the consultee will, it is hoped, provoke new possibilities.

---

Case study 4.1 An institutional example

The author was invited by a solution-focused colleague to join her to deliver a whole-day consultation to the senior management team (SMT) of a local authority secondary school. The management team of the school was relatively newly formed, with a new head teacher and a number of other new appointments. The team consisted of ten members. They were together facing a tough challenge in attempting to deal with a group of pupils who had been significantly disruptive, the school having also recently been viewed by OFSTED as 'in serious weakness', and facing reducing applications for places. The consultation day took place on the last day of the summer holidays before school was due to restart.

---

This account will detail the structure and the process of the day rather than the content of discussions. Focusing on the process of the consultation rather than the specific content of the discussions fits with the extent to which the solution-focused process is generic in its applicability. The particular nature of the issue being addressed does not determine the consultant's response, which is substantially unchanging in its overall shape regardless of the issue being addressed.

---

**Case study 4.1 contd.**

| Structure | Commentary |
|---|---|
| *Opening* | |
| • The consultants established and agreed ground rules, boundaries and arrangements for the day. | • The opening segment seeks to establish a purposeful working context. |
| • SMT members were invited to consider their best hopes for the day and in particular how they could know that their time, effort and energy had been put to good use. | • It seeks to indicate to the consultee that the consultant recognises that they come to the consultation with much already 'going right'. Focusing on what is going right and highlighting the fact that the SMT will wish to keep many things unchanged is also intended to reduce any anxiety about the consultative process. |
| Through feedback and discussion the group established and agreed how they could know that the day had been useful. | |
| • The consultants invited SMT members to discuss in pairs what they appreciated about the school and what was important to them to preserve and to maintain at a time when they would be challenged to change. | • The opening also seeks to highlight to the consultee that they will be 'in charge' of the process and that it will be the consultee who will commission the work, determining the direction as well as deciding whether the process was of use. |
| SMT members were invited to feed back to the whole group from their pairs discussions. | |
| *Preferred future* | |
| • SMT members were asked to: 'Imagine that a miracle has happened over the summer holidays and that when the students arrive the following day the SMT realise that the changes contained in their "best hopes" for the consultation have already been achieved and are already impacting favourably on school life.' They were then asked who would be aware of the differences. | • The detailing of the preferred future is a central part of the approach. The 'miracle question' is merely a device which allows consultees to suspend their hopelessness and to imagine the future as they hope for it, helping people to suspend their disbelief in the possibility of change brought about by their current state of 'problem domination'. The solution-focused consultant aims to invite |

*Continued*

The members of the SMT fed back who they felt would be the key witnesses of the change.

- The SMT was divided into three groups, allocated two key witness groups each, and asked to consider how these witness groups and how they themselves would know that the miracle had happened.
- Each group fed back, summarising their findings on a dry-mark board.

- The SMT was then asked to identify moments in the school's history that gave them hope that their preferred future for themselves and for the school was achievable.
- Members of the SMT then fed back to the group, being invited to specify, by the consultant, what it was about these moments that gave them hope.

- Members of the SMT were then asked to scale their confidence in the team's capacity to bring the 'miracle' into reality, with 0 standing for 'none at all' and 10 standing for 'total confidence'. Doing this in threes they were then asked to identify what they knew about the school, their students and themselves that contributed to the confidence that they already had.
- Quietly team members were then asked to reflect, privately, on what they might commit themselves to doing over the coming weeks that would contribute to their confidence rising one point up on the scale.

the consultee to imagine the preferred future in positive, concrete and observable detailed terms, identifying what will be the first small signs of progress towards this preferred state in the process. Imagining the future in these terms is associated with achieving it.

- Picturing the preferred future through the eyes of other key stakeholders helps the consultee to fill in the picture in detail, something also associated with good outcome.

- Remembering moments in the past that are congruent with the preferred future builds a sense of possibility in the consultee, and it is this specifically that is identified as the consultees describe what it is about those moments that give them hope.

- The scale is a useful way of concretising and consolidating a growing sense of confidence in change and of highlighting changes already achieved.
- Asking consultees to reflect privately on what they will contribute to the attempt to move forward allows each SMT member to commit the amount that is right for them without feeling pressured to commit to more than is realistic.
  Not knowing what others have committed to also allows the consultants to develop a sense of expectancy and a heightened interest in the subsequent contributions of others.

*Closing*
- Part 1
  The consultants then met, giving the consultees a break, and then returned to give feedback to the consultees on what they had learned during the course of the day which contributed to their confidence that the SMT could indeed work together to help the school to progress towards their aims and objectives.
  Consultees were then asked by the consultants to watch out for signs of progress in the school and to attempt to identify what seemed to be associated with progress being achieved. They were asked to watch out for what others were contributing that was useful.
- Part 2
  The consultants then met further after the end of the day and wrote to the SMT with further feedback about the basis for their confidence in the team, giving their evidence. The head teacher was asked to share this with the SMT.

- The feedback at the end of the meeting is intended to heighten the consultee's evidenced-based confidence that positive progress can be achieved, often citing signs of change already achieved as part of the picture.
- Asking consultees to focus on evidence of further change helps to build the experience of momentum whilst asking them to watch out for the contributions of others helps to foster a supportive and appreciative environment that is consistent with high morale and more progress.

*Follow-ups*
- Each follow-up session started with the question, 'What have you been pleased to notice since the last meeting?'
  Having identified signs of progress, the SMT were asked to discuss how these could be explained and who could be credited for contributing towards them.
- Further scale questions served to consolidate the progress made.

- Follow-ups highlight difference and seek to determine who and what can be credited for the progress and the changes that are being made.
  Each follow-up will end with the suggestion that consultees continue to look out for changes and what they notice their colleagues doing that is constructive and useful.

## Acknowledgements

I would like to acknowledge my discussions with Yasmin Ajmal, Chris Iveson, Di Iveson, Jane Lethem, Harvey Ratner and Denise Yusuf, all of Brief Therapy Practice, London, all of whom have shaped and influenced the ideas expressed in this chapter. In addition I would particularly like to acknowledge Maggie Stephenson, Educational Psychologist, formerly of Kent County Council, who jointly planned and delivered the consultation that is outlined in this chapter.

## Further reading

For those interested in reading more about solution-focused brief therapy, the most significant theoretical texts are those by Steve de Shazer (1985, 1988, 1991, 1994) with his book *Clues: investigations in brief therapy* (1988) probably the most accessible. For those looking for an introduction to the approach that is British-based, George *et al.*'s (1999) *From Problem to Solution* offers a clear and accessible description of the model. There is a range of texts looking at solution-focused brief therapy with children and adolescents (Selekman 1993, 1997, 2002; Lethem 1994) and a number of useful books examining the application of the approach with schools, including Rhodes and Ajmal (1995) and Ajmal and Rees (2001).

Specifically in relation to consultation there is very little written, although Thomas (1996), Triantafillou (1998) and Wetchler (1990) have discussed the use of the approach in supervisory work. The connections are, I think, clear and evident.

## References

Ajmal Y and Rees I (eds) (2001) *Solutions in Schools: creative applications of SF thinking with young people and adults.* BT Press, London.

Berg IK (1994) *Family-based Services: a solution-focused approach.* Norton, New York.

Berg IK and Miller S (1992) *Working with the Problem Drinker: a solution-focused approach.* Norton, New York.

Berg IK and Reuss N (1997) *Solutions Step by Step: a substance abuse treatment manual.* Norton and Wylie, New York.

de Shazer S (1985) *Keys to Solution in Brief Therapy.* Norton, New York.

de Shazer S (1988) *Clues: investigations in brief therapy.* Norton, New York.

de Shazer S (1991) *Putting Difference to Work.* Norton, New York.

de Shazer S (1994) *Words were Originally Magic.* Norton, New York.

de Shazer S, Berg KI, Lipchik E *et al.* (1986) Brief therapy: focused solution development. *Family Process.* 25: 207–21.

George E, Iveson C and Ratner H (1999) *From Problem to Solution: brief therapy with individuals and families.* BT Press, London.

Jacob F (2001) *Solution-focused Recovery from Eating Distress.* BT Press, London.

Lethem J (1994) *Moved to Tears, Moved to Action: brief therapy with women and children.* BT Press, London.

Lipchik E (1988) Interviewing with a constructive ear. *Dulwich Centre Newsletter.* Winter: 3–7.

Lipchik E (1994) The rush to be brief. *Networker.* March/April: 35–9.

McKergow M and Jackson PZ (2002) *The Solutions Focus.* Nicholas Brearley, London.

Rhodes J and Ajmal Y (1995) *Solution-focused Thinking in Schools.* BT Press, London.

Selekman M (1993) *Pathways to Change: brief therapy solutions with difficult adolescents.* Guilford Press, New York.

Selekman M (1997) *Solution-focused Therapy with Children.* Guilford Press, New York.

Selekman M (2002) *Living on the Razor's Edge: solution-oriented brief therapy with self-harming adolescents.* Norton, New York.

Thomas FN (1996) Solution-focused supervision: the coaxing of expertise. In: Miller S, Hubble M and Duncan B (eds) *Handbook of Solution-focused Brief Therapy.* Jossey-Bass, San Francisco.

Triantafillou N (1998) A solution-focused approach to mental health supervision. *Journal of Systemic Therapies.* **16** (4): 305–24.

Turnell A and Edwards S (1999) *Signs of Safety: a solution- and safety-oriented approach to child protection casework.* Norton, New York.

Walter J and Peller J (1992) *Becoming Solution Focused in Brief Therapy.* Brunner/Mazel, New York.

Weakland J, Fisch R, Watzlawick P *et al.* (1974) Brief therapy: focused problem resolution. *Family Process.* **13**: 141–68.

Wetchler JL (1990) Solution-oriented supervision. *Family Therapy.* **17**: 129–38.

White M (2000) *Narrative Therapy.* International presentation. Brief Therapy Practice, London.

# Chapter 5

# Social services consultation

*Angela Southall and Dave Poole*

## Introduction

This chapter describes regular consultation sessions at a social services area office over a five-year period. It presents a snapshot of the service, the various issues and concerns encountered and some of the uses made of consultation. It covers a range of consultations, from one-off case-related discussions to ongoing, regular consultation input to casework, and uses case examples to give a flavour of the work. A detailed account of ongoing case consultation is provided that outlines some of the social workers' experiences of 'being consulted to'. Consideration is also given to how consultation fits into the comprehensive range of child and adolescent mental health (CAMH) services and how it can be further developed.

## Why the tense relationships?

Social workers wishing to refer children to the community CAMHS teams often voice their dissatisfaction with what is felt to be a less than enthusiastic response. One of the main difficulties seems to be that of access and mutual expectations (Young Minds 2004).

Many access difficulties seem to arise from the low priority typically attached to social care referrals. Sometimes this is accompanied by a reluctance or even a refusal to accept referrals, on the grounds that the children's difficulties are being caused by 'social problems' rather than mental health ones. When help is sought to aid the planning process, there is invariably a refusal and a reiteration that the CAMHS remit does not include this type of work. At other times, social workers have found that there is a mismatch between their ideas of prioritisation and those of mental health workers. They have also found themselves frustrated by long waiting lists for CAMHS appointments at times when they see a family as requiring more immediate help. Some children, notably those looked after by the local authority, have found access to the community CAMHS particularly difficult. This has, in part, been explained by the traditional view that children needed to be in a settled placement before any therapeutic involvement could begin. Understandably, all of these things have led to frustrations on both sides.

A simple explanation of these difficulties is that health and social services have, for years, spoken a different language. Understandably, community CAMHS teams have more formal definitions of mental health than do social services and tend to construct their ideas around prioritisation on signs and symptoms of psychological distress. There is a necessary difference in focus and prioritisation between specialist CAMH and social services. For example, family breakdown, whilst distressing for everyone concerned, would not usually lead to a request for therapeutic help being prioritised. The community team would see this – some would say rightly so – as more of a social care emergency than a mental health one. Deliberate self-harm, on the other hand, would usually warrant immediate attention: a mental health crisis is indeed very different from a social care one. This fact alone goes some way to explaining some of the mutual frustrations felt by the two agencies.

Research suggests that professionals feel misunderstood by each other and it is this lack of understanding that they feel leads to inappropriate referrals – on both sides (Ackerley 2003). One might say that they look at the situation through two distinct lenses – one *social care* and one *health* – and then get cross with each other when they find that what they are seeing is different.

## Bridging the impasse

These difficulties have been long recognised (though not necessarily understood or given attention). They have begun to be addressed in recent years by the creation of interagency partnerships to deliver mental health services, for example specialist services for looked-after children. This reflects the developing imperative for 'joined-up' working, underpinned by legislation. Crises of confidence following high-profile tragedies have a depressing habit of occurring cyclically. When they do, they add further impetus.

## Emphasis on joint working

Research suggests that joint working is difficult to achieve and time-consuming (Sloper *et al.* 1999; Atkinson *et al.* 2001, 2002; Tomlinson 2003). However, joint working initiatives have also been shown to produce better outcomes for children, young people and families (Stobbs 1999; Sinclair 1998; Lloyd *et al.* 2001).

In recent years, Government policy has not only supported joint working but has in some cases placed a statutory duty on agencies to achieve it. Examples include the Children Act 1989, the Health Act 1999, the Crime and Disorder Act 1998 and the White Papers 'Modernising Social Services' (1998) and 'Modernising Health and Social Services – National Priorities Guidance' (1998). In 1997, the Secretary of State declared his intention to bring down the 'Berlin Wall' between health and social services, and in September 1998 the Government produced a consultation document, *Partnership in Action*, which proposed ways to facilitate joint working (Health Committee 1999). One of the key priorities in the joint social services and health agenda is to ensure that the two agencies work closely together.

The Quality Protects programme supports this agenda by aiming to achieve benefits for children in need of health, social care and education opportunities. The philosophy around integration also underlies the development of children's trusts.

## Professional and organisational cultures

In her survey of joint working, Beryl Ackerley (2003) makes a number of key observations, none of which are particularly 'new' but all are important enough to warrant repeating. She describes different organisational cultures and structures as presenting challenges to joint working, questioning the process and traditional time-frame of cultural change. She also notes the 'stark' contrasts in professional cultures between social services, education, health and the voluntary sector, with professional language not only excluding service users but also other professionals. Interestingly, she also articulates clearly the implicit (and sometimes explicit) hierarchy in joint working that most of us working in partnerships have long suspected (*see* Figure 5.1).

---

**Learning points**

- Different organisational cultures and structures present challenges to joint working.
- The organisational cultures of social services, education, health and the voluntary sector are in contrast.
- Professional language excludes service users and other professionals.
- There is a clear hierarchy in joint working.

---

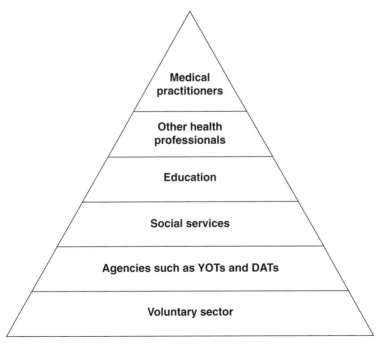

**Figure 5.1** Professional hierarchy (YOTs = Youth Offending Teams; DATs = Drug Action Teams).

## Consultation

It is clear that there has been considerable progress in the thinking around children's services. However, despite some headway being made on joint planning and prioritisation through links at the strategic levels, it often remains difficult to find the middle ground at the level of individual practice. Some interesting attempts to do so have been exemplified by interprofessional and interagency consultation. Here practitioners have not only ventured into no man's land together but have managed to explore the terrain (and even make maps).

Consultation can be described as a shared learning process and it is certainly the case that some of the learning has been about the things that do not seem to work. These warrant a closer look.

## Communication and consultation: how *not* to do it

Over the years, CAMH services have offered consultation to social workers in a number of ways, ranging from regular fora to individual *ad hoc* appointments. Anecdotal evidence suggests that such arrangements have not lasted and tend to 'fizzle out' after an initially good start. Sometimes they come to be seen as little more than gate-keeping exercises on behalf of CAMHS. This is probably not too far off the mark, in some cases. Similarly, the sense that the specialist CAMHS 'gateway' has been narrowed in response to growing demand is probably about right.

## Communication by proxy

Where community CAMHS teams have a social worker, the task of 'consulting' has been often given to him or her to do. Unfortunately, this has at times created mutual animosity, and is not without its sense of irony for field social workers who are left feeling that they are going round in circles and are being effectively refused access to 'real' mental health professionals. This attitude reflects the fact that the CAMHS social worker's status is seriously compromised if they are used – as many are – as a 'go-between': it can be difficult enough for them to have their mental health role acknowledged and appreciated. For instance, one very skilled community CAMHS social worker described her 'consultation' role to me as 'just gathering information' whenever a 'social services case' was referred.

The worst case scenario is that of the CAMHS social worker as a 'bridge' to social services in a way that also effectively ensures that no one else has to bother to develop any meaningful relationships (especially those who could really do with educating themselves). The bridge can become not only narrow but also more like a drawbridge, being pulled up again behind the social worker when they return to their 'home team'. In fact, it could be argued that the philosophy of 'having our own social worker in the team' is one of the powerful mechanisms that has allowed the health team to maintain a position of non-negotiation with social services.

## Alternative ways of offering consultation

Despite such potential pitfalls, some consultation fora have been set up differently and have been of perceived mutual benefit to both the recipients and the providers of the service. Incidentally, consultants may be drawn from a pool of mental health practitioners with a range of professional backgrounds (including, of course, social work); the difference is that they are about the real business of consultation. We shouldn't be surprised that people can tell the difference.

Real consultation is, essentially, about relationships. These relationships may be conceptualised as being organised around the problem for which consultation is being sought, including relationships between the consultee and their organisaton and that between the consultant and consultee. Within this context, the consultation becomes what has often been described as a process of mutual exploration and shared reflection. Importantly, consultation is not 'second best' to referring a case to someone else; sometimes it is 'first best', not only for the child and family but also for the worker.

## When consultation is best

There are many occasions when consultation might be a much better option than offering a direct piece of work. Some of these are given below.

---

Consultation might be best when:

- there is already a large professional system around the child
- work is currently being undertaken with the child/family that seems to be helping
- we might particularly want to give normalising messages about the child's perceived difficulties
- when a referral is the result of our own anxieties.

---

## When consultation leads to more work

Usually consultation can be effective in leading to less direct involvement by the consultant but this might not always be the case. It is not unknown to find oneself in the position of saying, 'I think this one needs to come to CAMHS', even when that might not have been the intention of the consultee. All consultants have the experience of something mentioned casually, almost as an aside, that rings alarm bells for them. Similarly, consultation can lead to more co-working and shared practice. It is certainly the experience of the author that consultation work is extremely demanding and frequently involves considerable involvement in the work of others. Consultation draws upon a different set of skills to those typically used by CAMHS professionals, or, at least, requires us to use them in a different way. Some of these things, hopefully, make themselves clear in the consultation work described.

## Consultation to a social services area office

The consultation mornings were set up to take place monthly at the local social services area office and include social workers from this and two other geographical areas. It was felt to be important to provide this service at base and not expect practitioners to travel to the CAMHS office for an appointment with a CAMHS worker. Some of the thinking behind this was that the consultations should be about building relationships and people would be more likely to get to know the consultant if she turned up at their office every month. There was also a sense of this being a more respectful way of doing things and, perhaps symbolically, that a clear message might be shared about consultation being focused on *their* work (their work – their territory, maybe). The mornings were organised by a social services administrator who arranged half-hour slots for each practitioner. This 'surgery' format was chosen by social workers, who wished to have confidential meetings with the consultant. The suggestion of group consultation was not taken up. From the start, the mornings were put to very good use with, typically, every bit of time used up. Unfortunately, the 'half-hour slot' format seemed to be quite resistant to change: this could be extremely challenging when several social workers might have two or even three families they wished to discuss during their half hour.

## Who uses consultation?

The example in Case study 5.1 is fairly typical of a referral to CAMHS that is followed through by a consultation meeting.

---

**Case study 5.1  The long-term 'heart-sink' case that has suddenly reached crisis point**

Helen, a new social worker in the area, rang the CAMHS office with an urgent request for an appointment for a family. She had recently taken over case responsibility following the departure of another worker. Unfortunately, she had taken over just as things reached crisis point for the family, culminating in court involvement. By coincidence, the consultant took Helen's call. She was requesting 'family therapy and behaviour therapy for one of the children and some parenting work'. The consultant discussed the case very briefly with the practitioner. After agreeing that the details of the request be faxed to the office, the consultant asked whether it might be helpful in the meantime to meet to discuss the case. This clearly came as a surprise to the practitioner, who, perhaps understandably, was concerned that this might mean her referral would not be acted upon. After some reassurance about this, there was an agreement to meet at the next consultation morning, which was three days away.

---

This request is somewhat typical of social services referrals to CAMHS, in that:

- the request is made at a time of high anxiety
- the treatment tends to be prescribed, rather than the concerns described (e.g.

'she needs post-abuse therapy' rather than 'she is having nightmares and has started bed-wetting').

During the consultation, the social worker described a very difficult situation in which she was involved in the assessment process of a mother and her five children. There had been longstanding concerns regarding neglect and abuse of the children. There was a particularly poor relationship between one child, Danny, and his mother and it was this child that had been the subject of physical abuse. The social worker outlined a catalogue of problems and, as she did so, the consultant thought she sensed both irritation at the consultation process and anxiety at the situation. She was able to comment on the pressure the worker was under to 'get things done'. She was also able to reflect the social worker's great anxiety and to validate this ('I can understand why you feel like this; the things you are telling me about are very worrying').

After much exploration, the social worker arrived at a position where she felt that none of the previous suggestions of what the family needed were appropriate. She had come to feel instead that the most appropriate course of action was to focus on the mother's ability to parent her children. Through further exploration, she was able to become clearer about her concerns for the children. She used the remainder of the consultation to focus on how she could proceed towards an assessment of the mother, as a prerequisite for any further work. Soon after this consultation, in fact, the consultant heard that care proceedings had been initiated.

## What use is made of consultation sessions?

A range of concerns has been brought to the consultation mornings. Most have tended to be individual case-based difficulties. Some of these have begun as 'referrals to be', like Helen's, already described. This was especially the case at the beginning of the service when there was, inevitably, an idea that this was the best way to get referrals 'accepted'. This happens much less nowadays but seems to be an important feature of the work. It has been important for the consultant to work with, rather than against, the practitioners who choose to use the session for a pre-referral discussion. What has proved essential, however, is that when this happens and it is agreed that the concerns warrant a specialist assessment (e.g. for autism spectrum disorder), the consultant passes on such information to the community CAMHS team, which ultimately makes the decisions about prioritisation and allocation of the case. In this way a clear boundary is maintained between the consultation forum and CAMHS, leaving the consultant freer to develop the distinct nature and purpose of the consultation forum. Similarly, if a request for a service is received by the community team that seems ambiguous or particularly complex, a consultation might be requested by the consultant in order to clarify concerns and to agree a way forward. Importantly, this is not routine; if it were, the meetings might be seen as just another means of CAMHS gate-keeping.

Consultation might start off as one thing and then become another (as in Case study 5.1) or might arise from a 'corridor conversation', as in the example given in Case study 5.2.

---

**Case study 5.2 The corridor conversation that becomes something else**

Lisa was an experienced social worker who had been based at the area office for some time. One day, she surprised the consultant by approaching her in the corridor and asking if she could teach her how to use a test that contributes to the assessment of attachment in children 'or, if you're not allowed to teach me, let me watch you do it'. A brief discussion followed and they agreed to meet the following day at the consultant's office, rather than wait a month for the next consultation morning.

---

At their meeting they explored together the details of the case and Lisa's involvement, with the consultant particularly focused on determining with Lisa what was the question she was wishing to answer. It emerged that she had been involved with the family over a considerable period of time. Things had got to the point where concerns about the children's future were being addressed. As part of this process, Lisa had agreed at a planning meeting to provide some feedback on the quality of attachments of one of the children. Having agreed to do this, she was anxious to make a start.

They agreed to a discussion of the many ways one might form an opinion about the quality of relationships in the family, without formal psychometric assessment. The consultant was interested in helping generate ideas of how Lisa could draw upon her own considerable resources and knowledge of the family to address this issue. It was agreed that there were three important components in enabling a full picture of relationships to emerge. The first of these was, inevitably, Lisa's knowledge of the family through her long period of involvement. Through this, she was able to have a sense of continuity, context and patterns of responding. Secondly, she could share her reflections and observations of the quality of relationships, maternal attunement and responsiveness to the child's physical and emotional needs. Thirdly, she could comment on the nature of the interactions between parent and child, as observed and recorded by her. On exploration, Lisa began to feel that such an assessment could not be, after all, as well achieved in a 'snapshot' and that a holistic view would be much more valuable. Although the consultant agreed to review the situation with her and to conduct a formal assessment of attachment if needed, in the event Lisa decided not to take this up.

## Notions of expertness

It could be said that both cases highlight similar issues. One of these might usefully be termed 'the impetus to act'. This seems to arise as a result of a combination of the nature of the case and the particular culture of social work that requires – often demands – that social workers intervene in some way. Sometimes, this intervention is prescribed by a manager, an 'expert' or even by court and serves to amplify the imperative to act.

Such processes militate against reflectiveness, whilst also denigrating skills. After I had seen Lisa, I asked myself, not for the first time, what it was that had stopped her using her skills in the first place. Certainly, court processes do not appear to recognise the expertness of social workers and social worker reports. There is a wider context, too, of professional culture expectations, of 'experts', and a general devaluing of social work skills and expertise. Added to this, it seems, is a day-to-day practice that is de-skilling and de-valuing. To the outside eye the agency context seems to be one of reactivity and to be subject to constant change – critical in generating helplessness amongst its workers.

## Reports for court

Having an awareness of some of these possibilities, it seemed important to the consultant to develop ideas with the practitioners that might begin to counteract some of the thinking around expertness. Court work seemed an obvious candidate for this and, to date, three different approaches have been tried, all with the aim of validating the practitioners' views. One of these has been to use consultation as a process that runs alongside the practitioner's assessment and reporting, so that when the report is produced it has been done so 'in consultation with' the consultant. In order to do this, the social worker and consultant met three times over a period of five months to discuss the assessment work and preparation of a report for court.

A second method has been for the consultant to write a letter, as distinct from a report, addressing the issues raised and directing parties, where appropriate, to pieces of work undertaken by the social worker (and duly the subject of their assessment report). Part of this process has been to articulate very clearly where the social worker is better able to address an issue, perhaps as a result of longer-term involvement and knowledge of the children and family. An example of this might be issues around family contact following adoption. In this way, the finished document becomes almost a joint report.

The third way, and for the consultant by far the best, is to try to support the social worker to intervene earlier in the process, so as to raise issues that challenge the need for an outside expert view. It has to be said that none of these have – yet – been all that successful.

To summarise so far, consultation mornings have led to a number of different types of consultation, as outlined below.

---

**Types of consultation**

- Consultation around a referral
- The corridor consultation ('Can I just run this by you?')
- Discussion of case work generally
- Discussion of a particular case
- Consultation on a specific report
- Continuous single-case consultation

---

The last one of these, 'continuous' case consultation on a single case, will be discussed in some detail below.

# Continuous single-case consultation

This type of consultation refers to a process by which the consultant is involved over a period of time in discussion about a particular case. In this instance, a case is described in which a social worker and family support worker worked with three children for 16 months. This process was punctuated by consultations with the author.

## The case of Katie, Hannah and Eliot

Social services initially became involved with the children following the murder of their mother by their father. There was a history of domestic violence, with the children trying to intervene to protect the mother. Maternal grandparents became the main carers for the three children who went to live with them. The children were 9, 7 and 6 years, respectively.

All children were, understandably, having difficulties coping. This was showing itself in very challenging and aggressive behaviours. The children also appeared objectively to be sad and confused. The grandparents were also grieving the loss of their daughter. Katie, the eldest of the siblings, had taken part in a counselling programme in an attempt to help her with her grief. Although this might have been helpful to her in a number of ways, it seemed to have no impact on her behaviour, which was of great concern.

Following a discussion with their team manager, the social workers sought permission from the family for a meeting with the consultant and, following this, for ongoing consultations.

At the first consultation meeting, the two workers, Emma and Dave, discussed their concerns. During this first meeting, much of the conversation was about Katie, who was seen as dominant, aggressive and bullying. However, exploration revealed considerable concerns about the other two children, Hannah and Eliot.

Hannah appeared to be the recipient of most of the aggression (from both siblings). She responded either by being withdrawn, quiet and moody or very attention-seeking. Hannah had recently started to act like an animal, crawling around on her hands and knees, saying she had given birth to kittens and carrying a toy kitten in her mouth. Her siblings had encouraged this practice, which they then used against her to cause embarrassment when people visited.

Concerns about Eliot centred around his physical aggression and destructiveness. Both workers doubted he was, as had been suggested, the least affected by the death of his mother and the subsequent loss of his father.

Finally, the workers, Emma and Dave, revealed something of their concern about the children's grandparents. The grandparents, both in their seventies, were in poor health. The grandmother appeared to be locked in her own grief and would seize every opportunity to discuss her daughter's tragic death. The grandfather reacted with frustration to this. Both grandparents frequently referred to Katie by her dead mother's name. They also commented regularly on how similar she was to her mother. These comparisons made Katie furious.

Additionally, Dave was immediately made aware of the difficulties raised for the family by him being male. He commented: 'My first visit to the family home proved difficult. There was no eye contact or communication; getting through the doorway was an achievement!'

There were so many issues here for the two workers to grapple with. In any situation like this it is easy to feel overwhelmed. One of them was to record later, 'How could we begin?' There are typically two responses to such feelings: the first is to feel inadequate and to want to give the case to someone else (maybe to a CAMH practitioner!); the second is to respond to an overwhelming feeling that you ought 'to do something' by finding a piece of work (either for yourself or someone else). To their credit, they did neither of these things. They did what is perhaps hardest of all, that is, they sought consultation to help them in their thinking about the work. At this point, one of the social workers commented: 'My description of my feelings at this point would probably be something like a workman who has a toolbox full of tools, but a fear of using them in case he gets it wrong.'

It is important to acknowledge the risk of being overwhelmed during the consultation process itself, given that the consultant is subject to those very same forces. The initial stage of our consultation process might best be framed as giving ourselves permission to feel the power of the things that threatened to over-whelm us. As a consultant to this process, my first task was to help the practitioners to resist the strong social work imperative to act: the first conversa-tions, I hope, helped them 'to be' rather than 'to do'.

We agreed to begin meeting to discuss the work that Emma and Dave were doing to help the children. Initially, meetings were scheduled for an hour a month but they would become less frequent as time went on.

At first, the main focus for the social workers was the children's behaviour. All three children were extremely challenging. Emma and Dave not only witnessed but at times were on the receiving end of their anger. The children were described as showing hatred and aggression towards each other and this had extended to those trying to help them. It was noted that the children appeared to be desperate for attention and love, to the point where they would physically attack workers who seemed to be giving attention to one of the other children. Emma and Dave had at first tried to initiate a regular programme of swimming. However, this was stopped as a result of the children's aggressive and dangerous behaviour towards them, namely, head butting, hitting and scratching, in addition to all three children joining forces to hold a worker's head under the water. Similar behav-iour whilst travelling in the car had also led to an agreement that any direct work or contact would involve two members of staff. It was noted: 'The three children display real hatred towards each other; this is not to be confused with sibling rivalry! They try deliberately to harm each other . . .'

## The first phase of consultation

The first 'phase' of consultations focused on exploring the meaning of the children's behaviour. Together, we thought about what might underlie their physical aggression. We thought about their angry and sad feelings and whether the angry feelings were sometimes effective at keeping the sad ones away. We thought together about how relationships might be in their family, where violence had been a feature; we wondered about love and intimacy and violence as attachment behaviours. We also shared ideas about the children letting us know through all of these behaviours just how frightened they were and allowing us to see all their frightening, mixed-up and messy feelings. The social workers had experienced how needy the children were and we began to see these behaviours as attachment-seeking, rather than attention-seeking, a plea to be loved and looked after.

The importance of boundaries and containment came to be emphasised through our discussions of the children's behaviour. If some of our guesses were right and these children were, indeed, feeling frightened and out of control, it was very important that their social workers, Dave and Emma, were able to maintain clear, firm boundaries and limits. This would help them to begin to feel safe again. Both workers had already begun to show that they could stick with the children's 'mess' and could cope with it. Through the process of joint exploration, we were also able to identify the workers' relationships with the children as being highly important. This was especially the case for Dave as he began to develop a relationship with them as a male who was not going to hurt them and who could be trusted.

This early stage of the consultation process can be summarised as follows.

---

**The first phase of consultation: exploration and clarification**

Focus on:
- the meaning of the children's behaviour
- the importance of boundaries and containment
- the importance of the workers' relationships with the children.

---

Dave has since commented on his feelings about taking up the consultation:

> When the consultations began, the arena for sharing, searching and sounding out was presented to us. Supervision was available through our team manager but I believe we required more, an understanding of how we were feeling, our emotions, the burden we were carrying and feedback to say we were making headway, or even if we were handling things badly. There is a need to know; we are dealing with people's lives and our actions could impact on the rest of their lives.

Alongside their work on limits and boundaries, Emma and Dave began a process of rewarding positive behaviour (not in any material way, but with their praise and attention – which was the most positive reward of all for these children). They established a long-term goal of returning to swimming.

This work was very hard-going. However, as Dave put it: 'Patience and perseverance paid dividends.'

## The second phase of consultation

The consultations were not broken down quite so distinctly into 'phases' as the description here implies. There were inevitably some overlaps and, at times, many things going on at once. This is real work, after all, not a textbook example! However, having made this point, it remains useful to conceptualise the consultation process as phases as this echoes the different areas of focus as the consultations progressed.

## What children tell us by their behaviour

Children tell us by their behaviour how they are feeling. By careful and thoughtful attention to this, we may also have a clue to some of the underlying processes. Where Katie, Hannah and Eliot were concerned, the fact that they began to accept boundaries and became less aggressive told us something about how safe they were beginning to feel with their workers, Emma and Dave, and that they were ready to move on.

Whilst still maintaining their strong, safe boundaries for the children, Emma and Dave felt the time was right to begin to encourage the children to express their feelings more. They had discovered that the older siblings liked to draw and discussed with the consultant their ideas for having 'drawing sessions' with the children, around which they could do some exploration of their feelings. Consultation therefore became the means of discussing these sessions and generating ideas together.

Emma and Dave decided to provide each child with their own folder for their drawing and to make the time for each child individually, as well as together.

Out of this work, they felt that much was achieved. The children were able to explore their feelings, particularly sadness and anger, and how they expressed them. They were also able to arrive at something of a resolution of their dilemmas around still loving their father (despite what he had done) and going on with life without their mother.

Again, their behaviour, during and after this work, is a key to understanding how they are managing their difficult feelings and, also, whether the work has been helpful. Although we might expect things to 'get worse before they get better', we would be hopeful of signs that things are being expressed and, ultimately, resolved:

> Working with the consultant, we were more confident with the situation. The strategies were in place and the way forward became illuminated, unlike the feeling of being in the shadows and searching for our way around, making an educated guess as to where we were heading.

Dave describes the work with the children becoming 'even more productive':

> . . . we were creating openings for discussion which led on to disclosure of feelings and emotions. A typical example was when the children were asked how they saw Emma and me. We were surprised when we were drawn on the large whiteboard as two angelic figures, complete with appropriate wings . . . A second example was the use of a drawing of a cliff with a person climbing; at the top of the cliff the rope was unattached and they were asked who would they trust to hold the rope. To our amazement, Emma and I were nominated.

From this, the workers were able to make guesses about how the children were thinking and feeling about them. This led to some exploration about trust and, in the consultation, some concerns on the part of the workers that they were now in a position where they might let the children down.

The content and graphic detail of the drawings had revealed vast quantities of information. Katie, the eldest of the siblings, drew pictures of all she had lost through death and the hope of things for the future that had died with her mother. At one particular stage she put herself in her drawing of relevant people or pets that had died. This promoted lots of discussion around her feelings of wanting to be in this particular place. Although the more outspoken of the family, Katie would not visit the death of her mum directly. Through her drawings, however, she began to talk about the death of her hamster and her mum's tragic death would begin to unfold around that. When the conversation reached that point, it seemed to Dave that they had permission to explore further. Dave and Emma used the children's responses to help them decide 'where to go next'.

They discussed with the consultant their ideas and 'guesses' about what all of these things might tell us about how the children were feeling and how they were making sense of their experiences. With the consultant, they explored how to begin to voice some of these things for the children through 'thinking aloud' about their guesses, giving voice to some of the children's feelings.

Dave describes how he and Emma have viewed their work with the children:

> The approach for each of the children is different, and their responses are individual. The whole family has moved forward towards some form of healing, each at their own pace and sharing their personal agenda with us.

---

**The second phase of consultation: helping**

- Helping the consultees to identify and celebrate their successes
- Helping to clarify strategies for keeping successes going
- Helping with the thinking and development of *their* ideas

---

The last point of the above is important. The work being described here is Emma's and Dave's – not the consultant's. This summary is not a 'how to' list, neither is it a description of what every practitioner might necessarily want to do: it is a description of how they did what they did, using consultation as a platform for their ideas.

## The third phase of consultation: consolidation and monitoring progress

Dave's and Emma's understanding of the children's difficulties had, from the start, included the wider family context. They had by now worked very hard with the children and established a position of trust with them. Alongside this had been a family focus. They realised that, irrespective of how much progress the children made, if they focused only on them the work would, inevitably, be 'undone', should issues at home remain unresolved. The children's grandmother, in particular, was described as 'stuck' in her grief, which meant that grief was more or less ever-present in the household.

Through conversations with Dave and Emma, the grandmother began to talk about her own feelings and to think about the relationships with grief that she, the grandfather and the children had. Out of this came a desire from her to pursue counselling in her own right. Contact was then made on her behalf with a support network that specialises in life after murder and manslaughter. The grandfather began to report positive changes, describing life as becoming much easier.

---

**The third phase**

- Reviewing progress made
- Exploring whether the necessary things are in place to sustain progress

---

### A long-term view

Dave has expressed an understanding that change for the children will be a long-term process. He acknowledges that there have been many changes in the children's lives and that confusion is still and will remain a dominant feature for them. He wrote recently:

> The work will continue for years to come, and as time passes unresolved issues will surface and have to be addressed.

What is interesting and, for the consultant, impressive is that Dave and Emma have somehow managed to resist the imperative to 'fix it'. Instead of pathologising the children's behaviour, they have sought to understand it and to support their process of change. They acknowledge that this is a long process and one that will, no doubt, continue for many years – hopefully without the need of a professional 'fixer'.

The work with these children was, in essence, about facilitating their healing. As Dave puts it:

> The ongoing work with the children has progressed greatly over the last year, and I firmly believe the underpinning of this progress has been the building of relationships and trust.

As for the children themselves?

> They now understand boundaries and adhere to them; they know it is okay to be angry, but it has to be channelled constructively. You can cry without being laughed at, and not all people are horrible; some people care and will help them learn to love and trust again.

## Conclusion

### What's the story?

People's problems exist in the minds of everyone thinking about them and are constructed by us as products of our agency and professional or therapeutic orientation. That is not to say they are not 'real' but that each one of us is responsible for creating a unique version, or story, of the problem, as well as contributing to a 'corporate' view of it. Consultation enables new stories to be constructed by providing an opportunity for safe exploration. The consultant is responsible for ensuring the safety of this journey: they must keep within the boundaries of territory that is manageable for the consultee and keep them both out of deep water. Furthermore, although the consultee is free to explore, the consultant does have a map and ultimately has a few ideas of where the best paths lie. They must feel comfortable taking the map out of their pocket if needed and not let the consultee lose their way.

The issue of containment is a very important one. All of us working with other people as professional helpers need, ourselves, to feel contained and 'held' through the helping process. For mental health practitioners this is usually done through clinical supervision. For the consultant, it seems that one of the most powerful and important factors in the consultation process is its containing function. For Dave, it was part of a wider support process. As he puts it:

> This case is extreme and I am part of a team. Consultation, supervision and guidance are given to me by the consultant clinical psychologist who specialises in trauma and loss, my team manager, and regular contact with the social worker who holds the case.

Consultation work can, however, reveal significant gaps in this support network. Often no teamwork is possible, owing to the scarcity of staff, and sometimes there seems to be no 'real' clinical supervision at all and no opportunity for space or time to reflect. These are symptoms of a system under stress. Unfortunately, they also perpetuate the stress. The problem for the consultant is that there is often nowhere to go with such observations. The challenge is to create somewhere.

## Why consultation?

Earlier in this chapter it was stated that consultation was not necessarily second best and, indeed, could be 'first best' in some cases.

It remains a myth that a complex problem needs a complex solution. You might say that this is the most powerful myth of mental health. Sometimes exactly the opposite is true. Many therapists and practitioners will admit to humbling experiences where a complex situation has been completely turned around by a very simple intervention at a practical level by a family support worker, classroom assistant or – horror of horrors – one of their own trainees! As professional helpers, we must be vigilant and watch out for the influence of this mythology of complexity, especially in ourselves. The author had a personal experience of this when consulting to a local children's unit and being told, on her first visit, about how 'clever' her predecessor was: the manager of the unit added, 'Of course, we didn't understand a word he said, but he was really good.' I try to remember this whenever I am tempted to be 'clever': ironically, I've noticed it tends to be when I'm not feeling it.

This chapter has sought to show some of the things that happen when practitioners for different agencies and backgrounds work together. The outcome for us was positive. New skills were developed – on both sides – which would otherwise have remained dormant. Also, the process has led to greater understanding and appreciation on the part of the consultant. As I write this, I realise the greatest learning curve has probably been my own.

In the longer case study described, that of Katie, Hannah and Eliot, it was possible to see how the children had been helped and supported through all their difficulties by two helpers who were clearly there to help the family – in a number of ways. Consultation meant that Dave and Emma could go on helping them: they did not have to become 'children with mental health problems' but could remain children in exceptional circumstances, who, in the end, became quite exceptional themselves.

## References

Ackerley BA (2003) *Towards Joint Working for Children and Young People.* Beryl.Ackerley@iow.gov.uk

Atkinson M, Wilkin A and Kinder K (2001) *Multi-agency Working: an audit of activity.* National Foundation for Educational Research, Slough.

Atkinson M, Wilkin A, Stott A *et al.* (2002) *Multi-agency Working: a detailed study.* National Foundation for Educational Research, Slough.

Health Committee Press Notice No. 3 of Session 1998–99, dated 13.01.99.

Lloyd G, Stead J and Kendrick A (2001) *Hanging On In There: a study of interagency work to prevent school exclusion in three local authorities.* National Children's Bureau, London.

Sinclair R and Vernon J (1998) *Maintaining Children in School: the contribution of social services departments.* Joseph Rowntree Foundation with National Children's Bureau Enterprise, London.

Sloper P, Mukherjee S, Beresford B *et al.* (1999) *Real Change Not Rhetoric: putting research into practice in multi-agency services.* Joseph Rowntree Foundation/The Policy Press, Bristol.

Stobbs P (1999) *Making It Work Together: advice on joint initiatives between education and social services departments.* National Children's Bureau Enterprise, London.

Tomlinson K (2003) *Effective Interagency Working: a review of the literature and examples from practice.* National Foundation for Educational Research, Slough.

Young Minds (2004) *Whose Crisis: access to CAMHS by other agencies.* Young Minds, www.youngminds.org.uk/magazine.

# Chapter 6

# Affirmation not treatment: consultation to women whose children have been sexually abused

*Michael Foulkes*

> ... I want to suggest to you that rape bears a direct relationship to all of the existing power structures in a given society. This relationship is not a simple mechanical one, but rather involves complex structures reflecting the complex interconnectedness of race, gender and class oppression which characterises that society. If we do not attempt to understand the nature of sexual violence and power, we cannot even begin to develop strategies that will allow us to eventually purge our society of the oppressiveness of rape.
>
> (Davis 1985, p. 9)

## Introduction

Sexual abuse is rape. The act is an abuse of male power over women and children. Although women sexually abuse children their number is small and their behaviour might be considered within the context of a society marked by male violence (MacLeod and Saraga 1988; Kelly *et al.* 1991). It will be argued that the trauma suffered by women whose children have been abused can only be understood by examining the 'complex interconnectedness of race, gender and class oppression' within a society divided by class and race and dominated by men. The tradition of critical theory will be employed to excavate the meanings hidden beneath the surface of the 'normal order' of things. Such an excavation will reveal the complex relationship between the endemic nature of sexual violence in our society and the suppression of this reality by restricting the problem of the sexual abuse of children to the pathology of the so-called 'dysfunctioning family'. The theory of the 'dysfunctioning family' rests on the assumption that the sexual abuse of children by their mother's partner is a consequence of marital dysfunction rather than an abuse of male power over women and their children.

An understanding of the relationship between the domination of men over women, sexual violence and the theorising of the 'dysfunctioning family' requires an appreciation of the concept of hegemony. In differentiating two types of political control, Gramsci (1966) contrasted the functions of domination (direct physical coercion) with those of hegemony (consent, ideological control).

**87**

Hegemony is the permeation throughout society of a system of values, attitudes and beliefs that support the established order or the ruling class. This 'world-view' is disseminated by the agencies of ideological control and socialisation into every area of daily life. It is so pervasive that the 'world-view' of the ruling class is accepted as being that of common sense. The success of hegemony is measured by the extent to which the ideas of the ruling class are accepted as being the natural order.

The term 'discourse' is associated with Foucault (1979, 1980, 1984) who sees discourse as those statements by persons and groups, such as psychiatry, the National Society for the Prevention of Cruelty to Children (NSPCC) and the law, who are accepted as having an authority to define or speak the problem. Foucault, by delving into the ideology of the established order, is extending the study of Gramsci to reveal the means by which power is promulgated and hegemony maintained.

Foucault's studies describe the rise of 'scientific' forms of social control by the authorities. The lives of individuals are to be strictly regimented. Foucault maintains that we are subject to power through truths that shape our lives and relationships. When discussing truths, Foucault is referring to constructed ideas that are accorded the status of being truths. These truths construct norms around which people are invited to construct their lives. Disciplines such as psychiatry, psychology and social work are described as being agents that penetrate society and subject people to the 'scientific' or 'normalising gaze'. Wise (1991) notes that the child abuse discourse does not include the voices of the main protagonists: abused children and their mothers, men who abuse and social workers. The child abuse discourse is dominated by those voices that speak the theory of the 'dysfunctioning family'.

What are the implications for social work of situating the sexual abuse of children in the realm of politics? How should social work address the position of women whose children have been abused by their father?

This chapter will discuss these questions by reference to the life of a woman whose children had been sexually abused by their father. What would she have seen reflected in the 'normalising gaze': a women who had allowed herself to fall in love with an abuser; a women who had failed as both a wife and a mother; a women who had failed to protect her children; a woman who deserved the condemnation of society; a woman who should fear the removal of her children from her care; a mother who should expect to be rejected by her children? And what of the other protagonists – social workers and other professionals – what do they see in the 'normalising gaze'? You must assume the compliance of the mother in the abuse of their child; you must always act in accordance with the principle that the interests of the children are paramount; you must be guided by the certainty inculcated by the child abuse inquiries and the proper use of the law?

This chapter is concerned with challenging the 'normalising gaze' that seeks to constrain and control, the 'medical model' that abrogates the authority to classify, assess and diagnose. It is the contention of this chapter that it is only by interrogating the 'normalising gaze', by understanding the politics of power, the advantage that power bestows, that we can begin to appreciate the trauma of a mother whose children have been sexually abused by their father or her partner.

## Social work, the state and hegemony

According to Yelloly (1980), the development of social work in England, Ireland, Scotland and Wales since the end of the Second World War has concerned itself with issues of training and professional organisation. A distinctive feature of this development has been the emergence of a professional ideology that has served to legitimise professional power and its exercise. The Beverage Report, the 1944 Education Act and emergence of the welfare state promoted the New Jerusalem of 'equal opportunity' in which poverty became a consequence of personal failure rather than a consequence of the structural causes of oppression inherent in society. Social work began to focus less on the structural aetiology of oppression and more on aspects of personality, which became the major aetiological factor of the 'dysfunctioning family'. Case-work was used to prescribe a distinctive approach to the problems of living in a capitalist society. Case-work, imported from the United States, was based upon psychoanalytic concepts that can be easily made to adapt to the requirements of a male dominated society. The resolution of the Oedipal Complex in boys, for example, through identification with the power and the authority of the father, ensures the perpetuation of patriarchy (Zaretsky 1976). As Eagleton says:

> The transition that Freud outlines, from an external parental agency to that introjection of it which is the superego, is parallel to the political shift from absolutism to hegemony, where the latter is understood as an internalisation of the law as the principle of one's own being.
>
> (Eagleton 1986, p. 275)

Thus, social work found itself compatible with the prevailing hegemony as it helped to ensure that the ideology of the ruling class was embedded in the self-conceptions of the individual. The concepts of psychoanalysis are appropriated by the ruling class to sanction an individualism by which people are removed from the context of class struggle. The tradition of social work has long reflected the tension between sociology and its commitment to an analysis that studies the interrelation of social parts and psychoanalysis that is concerned with investigating the unconscious and understanding the dynamics of the individual. Each of these disciplines contributes to our understanding of the complexity that is the human condition.

The public inquiries into the deaths of children known to their respective social services departments, from Maria Colwell (Department of Health and Social Security 1974) to Victoria Climbie (Laming 2003), have sought to reduce the problem of violence against children to a few pathological men, colluding women and incompetent social workers. Women are typically described as being 'fatally attracted' to violent cohabitees, a description that deflects not only from the issue of men's violence, but from the social and economic pressures upon women to remain with their partner (Parton and Parton 1989). The publicity attracted by these inquiries enables the 'good' family to distance itself from the 'bad' family and to conceal the possibility that problems associated with the parenting of children may derive from the 'normal' family relationships that obtain in society.

Wise (ibid.) asserts that the NSPCC, an institution frequently accorded the status of 'expert' by the media in matters concerning the protection of children, produces a depiction of child abuse that is consistent with the definition of abuse being a problem relating to the 'pathological family'. Such a portrayal disguises the endemic nature of sexual abuse and discourages a political critique of the male domination of society. Wise describes this depiction as being a product that is exchanged for the authority afforded the NSPCC by the media, particularly the tabloid press.

The position adopted in this study is one of understanding the discourse concerning the sexual abuse of children as being driven by the imperative that the endemic nature of male violence against women and children must be disguised by casting it as a problem relating to the supposed pathology of the 'dysfunctioning' family. Although the majority of sexual abuse is perpetrated by someone from outside the family (Kelly *et al.*, ibid.), theory and research has tended to focus on the abuse committed by the child's father or mother's partner. In defining abuse as a problem relating to 'pathological families', the abuse of children, according to Parton (1990), is removed from the realm of politics and placed in the hands of 'experts'. 'Experts' have access to an 'objective' and 'normative' knowledge that enables the assessment and diagnosis of those who are deemed to be deviant. The 'expert' is not interested in the 'others' story or perception of reality. Reality is reality as perceived by the expert.

Carole Ann Hooper's (1992) research with mothers of children who had been sexually abused by their father or mother's partner led her to the conclusion that the mother is the single most important person in her child's recovery, to the extent of her being described as the 'therapeutic parent'. To conflate the mother with the abuser is to seriously undermine her ability to recover from the trauma contingent on the abuse of her children. The task of the worker who meets with mothers whose children have been abused is to provide not treatment but a consultation that provides a secure base from which women are able to challenge the ideology implicit in the theorising of the 'dysfunctioning family', that finds women, as the non-abusing parent, complicit in their partner's abuse of their children.

## The knower and the known

At the end of 1988, the Minister of Health, David Mellor, introduced child protection guidelines to accompany the proposed Children Bill. The Department of Health's *Protecting Children: a guide for social workers undertaking a comprehensive assessment* would, according to David Mellor:

> . . . be invaluable to those training in social work because it sets out the basic principles of dealing with child abuse and offers a clear frame-work for assessing individual cases.
>
> (Department of Health 1988, p. 4)

McBeath and Webb interpret the manual as:

> . . . containing descriptives and prescriptives about the coherence and methods of implementation of child protection work which makes the individual social worker a cipher rather than an interpreter of the manual's recommended strategies. The text itself is a mode of profes-sional power that rationalises current knowledge of child protection

into a formulae for practice and reinforces a professional ideology by its attempts to exclude countervailing values, independent criticism and challenges to orthodoxy.

(McBeath and Webb 1991, p. 123)

The manual is informed by the ideology implicit in the theory of the 'dysfunctioning family' and fails to make any distinction between abusing and non-abusing parents. The manual appears oblivious of the position of power occupied by social workers in respect of their clients, the difference between the knower and the known. It is as though the worker is expected to be a colonialist whose mission in one of supplanting the economy, culture and even language of the indigenous population (Fanon 1967). The worker might be thought of as a researcher who generates knowledge that is used to ascribe meaning to the phenomenon of sexual abuse. The worker, however, is not encouraged to generate knowledge with their client but knowledge about their client, stripped of its social, economic and political context.

This knowledge is accorded the status of objectivity. As Edward Said writes:

> . . . the general liberal consensus that 'true' knowledge is fundamentally non-political obscures the highly, if obscurely, organised political circumstances obtaining when knowledge is produced.
>
> (Said 1985, p. 16)

In 1987, the family psychotherapist Gianfranco Cecchin published his paper 'Hypothesising, circularity and neutrality: an invitation to curiosity'. A reading of the paper suggests a connection between the thinking of Cecchin and the work of his compatriot, Gramsci:

> All behaviour, including language, is politically laden. Any particular action helps to organise and constrain the possible patterns of social intervention. Stated differently, our behaviour is always in relation to the behaviour of others – we 'act in relation'.
>
> (Cecchin 1987, p. 405)

The implication of this quotation is that psychotherapy is an intensely political activity. It is not possible to know the reality of another. We should only explore, together, in a spirit of curiosity, the logic of how we have adapted to the human condition, the prevailing hegemony, to those who have the power to define.

## The normalising gaze

---

**Case study 6.1**

Mrs Gregory, aged 26, has two children, an eight-year-old son named John and a six-year-old daughter named Lucy. A year previously, her son had told her that his father was sexually abusing both his sister and himself. Mrs Gregory immediately confronted her husband, informed the police and went, with her children, to live in a women's refuge.

---

Many women are unable to believe their children at the point of disclosure. Feminist researchers and practitioners such as Carol Ann Hooper (ibid.) and Christine Humphreys (1992) point to the considerable social pressures that would constrain women from believing their children: the loss of a partner; the under-mining of their status as wives and mothers; their sense of guilt at not knowing of the abuse and their failure to protect their children. Hooper and Humphries speak of women being in denial as a means of defending themselves from the trauma of the disclosure: their needing to find a security in which to begin the process of grieving the many losses contingent on their children's disclosure. Dwyer and Miller (1996), in talking of women's need to grieve their loss, draw on the work of Doka (1989) who refers to grief as being disenfranchised. Doka (ibid., p. 24) defines such grief as:

> . . . the grief that people experience when they incur a loss that is not or cannot be openly acknowledged, publicly mourned, or socially supported. The concept . . . recognises that societies have sets of norms – in effect 'grieving rules' – that attempt to specify who, when, where, how, how long, and for whom people should grieve.

Doka argues that grief may become disenfranchised for three reasons: the relationship between the grieved and the griever is not recognised, the loss itself is not recognised, or the griever is not recognised.

---

**Case study 6.1 contd.**

In Mrs Gregory's case, no charges were brought against the children's father, the Crown Prosecution Service advising that the children's evidence would not survive the adversarial rigour of the Court. Mrs Gregory confided:

> I promised them he would go to prison. I said daddy won't come back. He will go to prison for hurting you. They would not sleep by the window because he had told them that if they said anything he would come back and kill them and me. I promised them. But nothing happened.

---

In her children's eyes the failure to prosecute Mr Gregory confirmed their father's terrifying power. It denied both the children and their mother the affirmation they desperately needed in the face of his denial. It undermined their belief in their mother's ability to protect them. It served to reinforce the 'child abuse accommodation syndrome' (Summit 1983), the means by which the child tries to ensure their psychological survival by accommodating to the control of the abuser. Even in those few situations when the abuser is prosecuted, the child faces the difficulty that their story must be translated into a legal story, a necessity that produces a conflict between the therapeutic needs of the child and the legal needs of the Court (King and Trowell 1992).

The complexity and ambiguity of the 'therapeutic truth' is obscured by the need of the Court to have it translated into a legal story. In the telling of the legal story the child's experience is exposed. The control gained by the child in disclosing the abuse is undermined. The child is disadvantaged by the process of the legal system to the extent that its effect on the child is perceived as being a 'secondary abuse' (Richardson and Bacon 1991). Hooper (ibid.) points to the child's mother experiencing the Court's proceeding as an abuse by proxy. The Court is concerned with establishing the facts and finding the truth. It is not concerned with the truth of the devastating trauma suffered by the child and mother. Their trauma is subordinated to the legal procedures of the Court.

---

**Case study 6.1 contd.**

Mrs Gregory and her children were eventually rehoused to a 'hard to let' tenancy. A year following his disclosure, John told his teacher that his mother had hit him due to his being naughty. Mrs Gregory readily admitted that she had struck her son, adding that she could no longer cope with the behaviour of her children. Mrs Gregory agreed to her children being placed in foster care for the duration of the child protection investigation. The author was asked to provide an assessment of the children. Implicit in this request was the attribution that Mrs Gregory had caused her children harm. She was the subject of the investigation, not her partner who had abused his children. It was negotiated that the assessment of the children should include Mrs Gregory.

---

Hooper (ibid.) identifies that the support of women is a highly significant factor affecting the child's recovery, the absence of her support having significantly detrimental effects. The trauma experienced by the mother might be understood as being a secondary victimisation and her recovery does not necessarily match with that of her child. A child-centred focus can have the effect of dismissing the mother's trauma and increasing her sense of responsibility, failure and guilt.

The mother of a child who has been sexually abused by her partner suffers loss in several ways. The identification of women with the family means that the disruption of family relationships that the disclosure of abuse sets in motion may be intensely threatening. The expectation that the mother should be able to prevent harm to her child means that women are implicated in the abuse. Women whose children are abused by their partner are expected to choose between him and their child. The loss suffered by women whose children have been sexually abused must be understood in relation to a context in which the role of wife and mother are often the only occupations available to women (Parton 1990).

Mrs Gregory's rejection of support from the social services department, such as attendance at a family centre with the purpose of helping her to manage her children, might be understood as her need to deny the effect of her son's disclosure of abuse on her ability to manage her trauma. As with bereavement, the initial response is often one of denial. In the words of Mrs Gregory:

> I thought I was coping but now I realise that I was only pretending that everything was all right. It was too much to take on. Anyway, nobody

seemed to want to talk about it. It's disgusting isn't it? Who would want to talk about it?

---

**Case study 6.1 contd.**

Mrs Gregory had found her children's behaviour difficult to manage. Since the disclosure of the abuse her children had been arguing and fighting more often. She thought of this behaviour as being due to her inadequacy as a mother. She blamed herself for not knowing about the abuse. She had failed to protect them. She thought they were angry with her. She worried that they might no longer trust her. She felt rejected by them. Her husband had been a violent man, both verbally and physically. He constantly undermined her relationship with her children. She was told that she was not only useless in bed but that she was a useless mother. The children were afraid of him and would sit quietly in his presence.

Hester and Radford (1992) found that reaction to male violence includes self-doubt, self-blame, guilt, worthlessness, feelings of powerlessness and depression. Women tend to blame themselves for not leaving violent partners, even though allowing men to control them is often the only way of surviving the violence. As Mrs Gregory said:

> When I left him he said I would not cope, that my children would be taken into care. He said that I would plead to have him back. I am terrified of them [social services] taking the children.

---

Hooper and Humphreys (1998) draw on attachment theory in describing the debilitating effect that the trauma of sexual abuse has on the relationship between the mother and her children. Children, indeed adults, in times of stress and high arousal need the security afforded by proximity to their attachment figures. For the child recovering from sexual abuse the security provided by the non-abusing parent becomes crucial. By silencing the child the abuser denies him or her proximity and security. The abuser inculcates in the child the fear that they will be blamed by their mother. In times of anxiety a child needs the proximity of a parent who will protect and contain their distress. The abused child hesitates from telling their mother and, consequently, is left in a state of high arousal and anxiety: the containment so desperately needed by abused children is denied them and they find themselves alone in a prison of self-doubt and loathing. The most pressing need for the abused child and their mother following the disclosure of abuse is the rebuilding of their attachment. Mr Gregory told his children that he would kill their mother if they were to say anything. Mrs Gregory was deeply troubled that her children seemed unable to confide in her when they were first abused.

Miller (1995) suggests that the mothers of abused children often play out an unconscious wish to be punished for the sense of failure attendant on the disclosure of abuse. Mrs Gregory's injury to her son might be understood as a means by which her need to be punished would be realised by the removal of her children from her care. The injury might be understood as her attempt to alert the social services that she was not coping with the trauma of the abuse without consciously recognising that the trauma was threatening to overwhelm her psychological resources.

Mrs Gregory commented:

> I thought they [social services] would have asked about my relation-ship with my husband. I thought they would want to know why I had married him. I didn't know he would hurt his children when I married him. But somehow I can't stop thinking that it must be my fault.

Mrs Gregory gave several indications that she feared being blamed for the abuse of her children. The disclosure that her children had been sexually abused seemed to have led to her questioning every aspect of herself. It was as though she had been taken to that place in her mind that is the repository of all our failures, sins and shame, a place resembling a black hole from where it feels impossible to escape.

---

**Case study 6.1 contd.**

Mrs Gregory said that she could not bear to touch her son, explaining that her husband had done things to him that he had done to her in bed. She worried that her son would perceive her not touching him as meaning that she hated him. She worried that he might have regretted having said anything about the abuse. She was worried by these thoughts and feelings. She felt diminished by her general practitioner's dismissal of her disturbing dreams, especially one in which she was masturbating in front of her son, as being no more than sexual fantasies. She was frightened by her anger towards her daughter. She found herself asking why Lucy had not stopped him, why she had not told her mother. Had her daughter instigated the abusive relationship and had she, as her father claimed, enjoyed it?

> I did love him. I don't anymore. I can't understand women who have them back. People don't understand how much it all means. He was my backbone. He looked after me. And then I hated him. I was saving my wedding dress for Lucy. That's shredded. I have cut him out of all the photos. He's dead now. It is as though someone had died. We needed for nothing. Now all that has gone.

---

It seems that it was only following the injury that she had inflicted on her son that Mrs Gregory allowed herself to acknowledge her pain. It was as though she had been in denial of her need to grieve. To have acknowledged this need would have been to acknowledge the permanence of what had happened.

Children will avoid talking about the abuse to their mother until they are confident of their mother's ability to manage the experience of telling. It is crucial that attention is given to the mother's need to grieve following the disclosure of abuse. The mother needs a safe place, a place where she feels held, metaphoric-ally, and contained, if she is to hear and respond to her child's story.

In the context of sexual abuse, mothers are described as being the most significant actors in the protection of their children (Hooper, ibid.). They are more likely than professionals to be told of the abuse. When professionals do become involved, the decision as to whether to remove children from home depends on the ability of their mothers to protect them from further contact with the abuser.

## The concept of containment

The concept of containment, as developed by WR Bion (1970) in his concept of the 'maternal reverie', is the ability of the mother to receive, take in and hold her infant's hostile and destructive feelings, feelings that the infant experiences as persecutory (*see* Chapter 3). The ability of the mother to hold these feelings or projections without perceiving them as an attack on herself prevents the infant from becoming overwhelmed by feelings of anxiety. The ability of the infant to put or project their 'bad feelings' into the mother is a necessary defence against anxiety that if not contained can constrain their psychological development. The infant's experience of their mother's ability to hold their ambivalent and conflicted feelings enables them to feel 'held' and allows for the gradual taking back and integration of their hostile and persecutory feelings.

Mrs Gregory might be thought of as being required by her children to receive and hold their need to evacuate themselves of the messy feelings contingent on the abuse by their father. The mother's ability to hold her child's projections, rather than experiencing them as attacking and then retaliating, contributes to the child's sense of being contained. It is as though Mrs Gregory's children were saying: 'You hold onto our bad feelings that are a consequence of our father abusing us until we are able to sort them out. For the time being we need to put all the feelings we cannot cope with into you. We're sorry.'

It is doubtful that Mrs Gregory could have held her children's projections without her being left with a sense of persecution that would have intensified her feelings of failure and guilt at her son's disclosure of the abuse. In order to provide her children with the experience of feeling contained, Mrs Gregory needed to feel contained by her worker, to find a safe place in which her projections could be held until they had become sufficiently detoxified for her to accept their return. We all need the proximity of a secure base from which to venture forth on our journey to explore both our inner and outer worlds (Bowlby 1965).

The concept of containment is extended to include the relationship between the social worker and their supervisor. The absence of this containment can leave the worker without the means of processing their feelings. This allows for the possibility of the worker retaliating through 'acting out' their unprocessed material that has emerged in response to the client's story.

## Social work organisations, anxiety and defence

A central dilemma in the profession of social work is how to accomplish the task of protecting children whilst enabling as many children as possible to continue living with their family. This role is highly ambiguous, an ambiguity that propels social workers into a desire for certainty.

Morrison (1991) contends that social workers expect to experience stress generated from the work they undertake but are far more distressed by the secondary stress arising from the agencies' response when this happens. Morrison offers a theoretical framework in the form of the 'professional accommodation syndrome', in an attempt to explain the damaging effects of secondary stress on workers. Morrison's model is an adaptation of Summit's (ibid.) 'child abuse accommodation syndrome'. Workers are trapped in a paradox whereby telling the truth about their feelings is seen as being unprofessional and maintaining the lie is seen as coping. The accommodation is made by their deciding that the fault lies with them for feeling as they do. If they were a better professional or person it would not happen. Professional systems can develop into abusive systems whereby the worker is at the receiving end of the enormous social anxiety generated by the realisation of the extent of abuse within our society. It is as though society and their own organisation are waiting to blame them for any error of judgement (Jones 1991).

A psychoanalytical perspective within organisations suggests that behaviour is motivated by a need to contain anxieties that threaten to overwhelm. Menzies-Lythe (1988), for example, suggests that there is a complex of early life anxieties concerning death and sexuality in the nurse's daily work:

> Nurses are confronted with the threat and reality of suffering and death as few lay people are. Their work involves carrying out tasks, which by ordinary standards are distasteful, disgusting and frightening. Intimate physical contact with patients arouses strong libidinal and erotic wishes and impulses that may be difficult to control. The work situation arouses strong and mixed feelings in the nurse: pity, compassion and love; guilt and anxiety; hatred and resentment of patients who arouse these strong feelings; envy of the care given to the patients.
>
> (Menzies-Lythe 1988, p. 46)

Menzies-Lythe suggests that nurses defend themselves from the anxiety associated with these 'strong feelings' by employing 'social defences' that enable them to distance themselves from their patients. An example of such 'distancing' is the reference to patients by their type of disease.

Similarly, it is not surprising that social workers who are working with children who have been sexually abused should feel '. . . strong and mixed feelings . . . pity, compassion and love; guilt and anxiety; hatred and resentment of patients who arouse these strong feelings; envy of the care given to the patients' and seek to displace these disturbing feelings on to their clients who then become the problem (Bion 1961). The insistence that the abuse of children can be predicted and managed by recourse to check-lists, supervision and 'proper' use of the authority of the law, the seductive simplicity of the theorising enjoined in the 'dysfunctioning family', and the belief that it is possible for the therapist to know the reality of the family conspire to form what Mason (1993) describes as being an 'unsafe certainty', in which the certainty of the worker denies the client the opportunity to tell their story. The worker assumes the normalising gaze.

---

**Case study 6.1 contd.**

The 'assessment' of Mrs Gregory comprised four meetings. The first meeting was with Mrs Gregory alone. The meeting was marked by the pain and anguish she endured as she struggled to tell her story. The author listened and sought to affirm her experience. The subsequent two meetings were with Mrs Gregory and her two children. The children were encouraged to speak of their stories in the presence of their mother. The children were helped by their mother and the author to disentangle the distortions that the behaviour of their father had produced between them and their mother. Their feelings of love and anger for their father were spoken. They were held in their mother's arms as they grieved the loss of their father. She helped them to understand that they were not responsible for what had happened. They had embarked on the process of relinquishing the survival mechanisms they had adopted to survive their trauma, a process necessary for them to become children again. The final meeting with Mrs Gregory was memorable for the confidence with which she reviewed the process by which she had freed herself of the role of victim. John and Lucy were returned to her care.

---

## Conclusion

Social work is not a neutral activity. The ruling class would have us believe otherwise. Social work, in the view of Althusser (1969), is an agent of state control. Its legitimate purpose is to perpetrate a view of society that accords with the need of the ruling class to disguise the violence that maintains its domination. The study of sociology forms part of the bedrock in the education of the social worker. This tradition invites us to adopt a critical approach to social problems such as the sexual abuse of children. As social workers we have a duty to interrogate the theories on which our practice stands. Whose purpose does the theory of the 'dysfunctioning family' serve? In what ways does this theory construct a particular view of women as mothers? Who benefits from this construction?

It is essential to the recovery of women whose children have been sexually abused that we should be aware of the danger of replicating the abuse of power that these women have already suffered. Women who are able to believe their child's disclosure reclaim a measure of control from the abuser. This control is easily undermined by a response from agencies that fails to differentiate between the abusing and non-abusing parent, a response that locates the woman as colluding with the abuser.

If the mother is to assume the role of therapeutic parent she needs a safe place from which to begin her painful journey to recovery. This safe place can be provided by the worker whose ability to empathise with the mother is informed by an understanding of the political oppression of women. This understanding becomes available to women whose children have been abused through the presence of the worker, empowering them to challenge the 'normalising gaze'. As Mrs Gregory said:

It was weird in a way. In a sense, to get you to see the light you've got to talk about everything that put you there, in the darkness. You can't just sit there on your own and think about these things. You can't do it, you only get worse. Just by talking with someone, by realising that it's not you, it's not your fault, you feel stronger.

# References

Althusser L (1969) *Lenin and Philosophy*. New Left Books, London.

Bion WR (1961) *Experiences in Groups and Other Papers*. Tavistock, London.

Bion WR (1970) Container and contained. In: *Attention and Interpretation*. Tavistock, London.

Bowlby J (1965) *Child Care and the Growth of Love*. Penguin, London.

Cecchin G (1987) Hypothesising, circularity and neutrality: an invitation to curiosity. *Family Process*. **26** (4): 405–13.

Davis A (1985) *Violence Against Women and the Ongoing Challenge to Racism*. Kitchen Table/ Women of Color Press, Latham, NY. Quoted in: MacLeod M and Saraga E (1988) Challenging the orthodoxy: towards a feminist theory and practice. *Feminist Review*. **28**: 10–56.

Department of Health (1988) *Protecting Children: a guide for social workers undertaking a comprehensive assessment*. HMSO, London.

Department of Health and Social Security (1974) *Report of the Committee of Inquiry into the Care and Supervision Provided in Relation to Maria Colwell*. HMSO, London.

Doka K (1989) *Disenfranchised Grief: recognising hidden sorrow*. Lexington Books, New York. Quoted in: Dwyer J and Miller R (1996) Disenfranchised grief after incest. *Australian and New Zealand Journal of Family Therapy*. **17** (3): 137–45.

Dwyer J and Miller R (1996) Disenfranchised grief after incest. *Australia and New Zealand Journal of Family Therapy*. **17** (3): 137–45.

Eagleton T (1986) *The Aesthetics of Ideology*. MacMillan, London.

Fanon F (1967) *The Wretched of the Earth*. Penguin, London.

Foulcault M (1979) *Discipline and Punishment: the birth of the prison*. Peregrine Books, Middlesex.

Foucault M (1980) *Power/Knowledge: selected interviews and other writings*. Peregrine Books, Middlesex.

Foucault M (1984) *The History of Sexuality*. Peregrine Books, Middlesex.

Gramsci A (1966) *The Prison Letters*. Pluto, London.

Hester M and Radford L (1992) Domestic Violence and Access Arrangements for Children in Denmark and Britain. *Journal of Social Welfare and Law*. 1: 57–69.

Hooper CA (1992) *Mothers Surviving Sexual Abuse*. Tavistock/Routledge, London.

Hooper CA and Humphreys C (1998) Women whose children have been sexually abused: reflections on a debate. *British Journal of Social Work*. **28**: 565–80.

Humphreys C (1992) Disclosure of child sexual assault: implications for mothers. *Australian Social Work*. **45** (3): 27–35.

Jones E (1991) *Working with Adult Survivors of Child Sexual Abuse*. Karnac Books, London.

Kelly L, Regan L and Burton S (1991) *An Exploratory Study of the Prevalence of Sexual Abuse in a Sample of 16–21 Year-Olds*. Child Abuse Studies Unit, Polytechnic of North London.

King M and Trowell J (1992) *Children's Welfare and the Law: the limits of legal interventions*. Sage, London.

Laming Lord H (2003) *The Victoria Climbie Inquiry*. HMSO, London.

MacLeod M and Saraga E (1988) Challenging the orthodoxy: towards a feminist theory and practice. *Feminist Review*. **28**: 10–56.

Mason B (1993) Towards positions of safe uncertainty: human systems. *Journal of Systemic Consultation and Management*. **4**: 189–200.

McBeath GB and Webb SA (1991) Child protection language as professional ideology. *Social Work and Social Services Review*. **2** (2): 119–29.

Menzies-Lythe I (1988) *Containing Anxiety in Institutions: selected essays*. Free Association Books, London.

Miller A (1995) *The Drama of Being a Child*. Virago, London.

Morrison T (1991) *Staff Supervision in Social Work*. National Society for the Prevention of Cruelty to Children, London.

Parton C (1990) Women, gender, oppression and child abuse. In: The Violence Against Children Study Group. *Taking Child Abuse Seriously: contemporary issues in child protection theory and practice*. Unwin Hyman, London.

Parton C and Parton N (1989) Child protection: the law and dangerousness. In: Stevenson O (ed.) *Child Abuse: professional practice and public policy*. Harvester Wheatsheaf, London.

Richardson S and Bacon H (1991) A framework of belief. In: Richardson S and Bacon H (eds) *Child Sexual Abuse: whose problem?* Venture Press, Birmingham.

Said E (1985) *Orientalism*. Penguin, London.

Summit R (1983) The sexual abuse accommodation syndrome. *Child Abuse and Neglect*. **7**: 177–93.

Wise S (1991) *Child Abuse: the NSPCC version*. Feminist Praxis, Manchester University.

Yelloly M (1980) *Social Work Theory and Psychoanalysis*. Van Nostrand Reinhold, Southampton.

Zaretsky E (1976) *Capitalism, The Family and Personal Life*. Pluto, London.

# Chapter 7

# Consultation in child and adolescent mental health services

*Rajeev Banhatti and Kedar Nath Dwivedi*

## Introduction

The word 'consult' originates from Latin, meaning to 'take counsel'. This basically means taking advice. The term 'consultation' has been used in various different contexts and with different meanings and is in danger of becoming meaningless and ubiquitous like the word 'depression'. In this chapter it is used to describe the process of seeking *expert* advice, which is usually an *indirect* way of helping a patient, client, student or a consumer, depending on whether the consultee is a doctor, psychologist, therapist, teacher or social worker.

The authors will go on to look at the uses of consultation in the context of contemporary child and adolescent mental health services (CAMHS). Looking at specific contexts in which consultation can be offered by a mental health professional based in CAMHS will follow this. As both authors are child and adolescent psychiatrists, the emphasis will be on psychiatric consultation. However, most of the principles and almost all of the content should be applicable for any reasonably senior mental health professional, irrespective of the discipline that they may come from. At present this may mean a consultant psychologist, a nurse consultant or a consultant psychotherapist.

Consultation is similar to but different from giving general advice, supervision or counselling as clarified elsewhere in this book. In context of CAMHS, it should mainly be contrasted with direct assessment and case management. However, in the real world often boundaries between consultation and other activities become blurred and there is a clear overlap. It is useful to reflect upon such occurrences before 'consultation' becomes so eclectic that it loses any specificity. Sometimes consultation can lead to the consultant or another team member taking on a different task, such as assessment or case management.

## Uses of consultation

Uses of consultation include:

- reaching out indirectly to more children and young people in need through professionals working with them directly
- empowering professionals in using strategies to improve the mental health of children
- the learning of new skills or practising newly learnt skills

- enabling the consultee to feel more confident about doing the right thing and not overlooking obvious risks
- helping to develop a common language about child mental health and ill health
- reducing inappropriate referrals to CAMHS and making service provision more cost-effective and efficient
- allowing for the consultant child psychiatrist to have direct involvement with only the more complex or persistent problems after initial interventions by other professionals have been tried.

## Before you begin

There are many traps for the unwary that should be avoided before embarking on offering consultation to another professional.

When consultation is offered but the referrer is expecting more traditional direct assessment and treatment, it can lead to a sense of disappointment. Therefore one needs to explore the referrer's expectations and why there might be different views about the appropriateness or inappropriateness of consultation. When an agreement cannot be reached it is often advisable to give the referrer the benefit of the doubt and see the case. If similar dilemmas keep arising with the same practitioner it might be helpful to meet them, preferably in their working environment, in order to try to make sense of their predicament. This may sometimes bring forth managerial or organisational issues (often about funding and resources) that warrant negotiation at the managerial level.

In one of the author's teams, a senior nurse has successfully piloted a project to deal with referrals with unclear expectations, exploring the role of specialist CAMHS in service provision. She takes all such referrals from the weekly meeting and contacts the referrer to clarify their expectations. This has sometimes led to telephone consultation followed by closure or to a screening assessment to further clarify the role of CAMHS. This project has been helpful in reducing the waiting list for specialist assessment and intervention and has also been replicated in another team. It might be expected that managers would be interested in funding posts which have consultation, screening and education of tier 1 staff as the main components of the job description.

If referrers in a particular locality demand more direct assessments, it is preferable that senior staff address this as a managerial issue. The person with managerial responsibility is in a position to educate commissioners about the resources required to meet such demands: these are conceivably much greater than are currently available to most specialist CAMHS in the United Kingdom. If this is not forthcoming then the referrers need to be educated in new ways of working with specialist CAMHS. It is probably crucial that the referrers, commissioners and managers communicate and meet often to synchronise their efforts to develop services that satisfy local population needs. Consultation/liaison can provide an opportunity to link in with the process of service development.

It is useful to reflect on a number of issues when a consultation is requested. Some of these are given in Box 7.1.

Box 7.1 Helpful consultation questions

- What is the problem for which I am being consulted?
- Do I have the expertise to offer consultation about this specific problem?
- If I do not have the expertise but a colleague does, can I arrange a consultation meeting with that colleague?
- Will it be more helpful to arrange a joint meeting with the colleague and consultee?

Case study 7.1

A 12-year-old boy had been referred as an urgent case by a social worker to a multidisciplinary CAMHS team. The social worker had requested a psychiatric assessment and appeared angry from the letter that this had not been done. The child had been in care from an early age and had been resident in a therapeutic community for four years. The social worker was invited for a consultation to the team's meeting. It became clear that the social worker was probably the only person that the child had known with any continuity for three or four years and she was acutely aware of the anger that the child was thought to be experiencing as a result of serial abandonments. The child had been sexually abused early on in life by an older adolescent and had also been rejected by his mother. The social worker wondered whether he had psychopathic traits or organic problems and whether his inappropriate, clingy, often sexualised behaviour was indicative of a psychiatric disorder. She was also angry that the child had been sent back into foster care and to a special school from the therapeutic community without proper planning.

On reflection, the social worker realised that she herself was ambivalent about the conflicting needs of containing the child's behaviour as opposed to letting go to see how he handled responsibility for his behaviour in the outside world. There was one senior child psychiatrist present in the meeting who had considerable experience of working with looked-after children and attachment issues. He felt that the social worker should continue her relationship with the child as she was by now the main attachment figure for him. One of the authors offered consultation to her to explore concerns about the child's mental health. This was done by means of discussion, using check-list criteria and reviewing the child's mental health file. Together, the consultant and social worker were able to reach the joint conclusion that it was very unlikely that the child had a primary developmental disorder or a conduct disorder. In addition, the consultant arranged a meeting with a psychologist colleague with special responsibility for offering consultation to professionals dealing with looked-after children. This process proved satisfactory to the social worker.

This exercise in itself reduced a great deal of administrative time and possible conflict that would have come about if the team had simply sent a letter to the social worker asking more questions or refusing the referral as being inappropriate. Perhaps even more importantly, the shared process of exploration and negotiation was beneficial in facilitating greater mutual understanding between the different agencies and improving the potential quality of communication for the future.

## Putting theory into practice

Quite often an idea can look very appealing in theory but can prove to be very difficult to convert into practice over a period of time. Consultation projects can often start with a bang, only to go out with a whimper within a few months. Hence it is important to plan well before starting consultation as a regular individual or team activity. It is important to allocate ample time for consultation and to keep a record of consultations offered. It is all too easy to get into a lot of important work through consultation without creating enough space and a system of documentation.

A practitioner can initially negotiate one weekly session for consultation. In the early days this can be split into different activities, such as telephone consultations, drop-in consultations and a record kept of consultation activities done during the week. The budding consultant should accept that, like most new skills, this one will also feel quite difficult to begin with but will become second nature as they become more confident with practice. It is important to realise at the outset that the session can be structured and restructured to suit the needs of consultees within the bounds of what the consultant can provide within a given time-frame. The documentation helps by providing factual information which can be crucial in reflecting on future needs, parts of audit, research, clinical governance and appraisal activities.

## Consultation in a multidisciplinary team

A child mental health professional offering consultation needs to have a fairly deep, theoretical and experiential understanding of group processes to withstand the rigours of being a consultant in a multidisciplinary team. A number of authors have already commented on the importance of resisting the temptation of being the expert who knows all answers or one who can rescue others in all situations. Sometimes this can be effective in the short term but can disempower other professionals in the team and turn the consultant into a scapegoat when the team is under pressure, or when something has gone wrong with a particular case. The consultant should try to remember which hat they are wearing as professional expert and then try to actively listen to the problem, ask for more information and use the model of consultation that feels appropriate and familiar. The consultee – and not the consultant – should choose the course of action and also clarify expectations from the consultation at the outset. It is important to determine whether the consultee is satisfied with the outcome of the consultation. If not, another consultation should be arranged to explore the reasons for any dissatisfaction.

The consultant should keep in mind not only the medical, psychological and social aspects of the assessment but also the risk assessment element in every case.

They should not be hesitant about taking control of a potentially risky situation but should make the shift from consultation to case management with a clear awareness and explicit agreement of the consultee.

## Content, process and context

The content of consultation can vary from a reflective dialogue, to exploration of the meaning behind the problem for which consultation has been requested, to advice about the options of further assessment or management of a particular child. CAMHS have gone through many rapid changes in the last two decades and the context illustrated in Figure 7.1 can change over time depending on the national and local initiatives. However, the basic process of consultation will involve a child mental health professional with expertise of a generic or specific nature offering advice to another colleague working with a child in a similar or different setting. At present the specialist child mental health professional usually operates at a tier 2, 3 or 4 level of service, but the work of consultation could take place in any setting. CAMHS appear to be following the developments that adult community mental health services experienced in the early 1990s and more and more consultants are allocating professional time to work at the primary care (tier 1) level to offer a more timely consultative service. New posts of primary mental health workers (PMHWs) or nurse consultants are becoming increasingly common, where a large part of their job descriptions constitutes consultation to tier 1 services. In Figure 7.1, bi-directional arrows between the boxes indicate the flexible working among multidisciplinary CAMHS teams. There is an element of peer supervision as well as mutual consultation built in among team members in this model of working. Most practitioners inside the circles are usually based within tier 1 services at present.

The tiered model of CAMHS (NHS Health Advisory Service 1995) replaced the previous model, which described services in terms of primary, secondary and tertiary care. In the authors' opinion it is better suited to encapsulate the complexity of CAMHS. However, the flexibility it offers in thinking of the tiers as abstract concepts simultaneously referring to a particular set of service process,

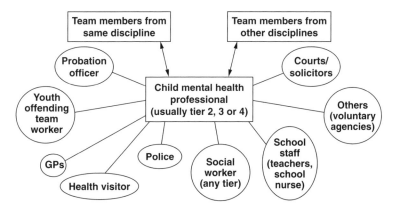

**Figure 7.1** Consultation in contemporary CAMHS.

level of professional expertise and demographic location has to be combined with specificity to clarify professionals' roles.

## Consultation in the primary healthcare setting

Prevalence of mental health problems in children and adolescents seeing their GPs has been found to be as high as 25–40% (Kramer and Garralda 1998). Only 2–5% of these present with emotional or behavioural disorders *per se* (Kramer and Garralda 2000). The rest present with somatic or social symptoms. Recognition of psychiatric disorders by general practitioners (GPs) is limited and the rate of referral to CAMHS can be approximately 3% or even lower. There is some evidence that shifting to a consultation–liaison style between community mental health teams and general practice is a double-edged sword. It can lead to an increase in the number of referrals (hardly an incentive for already overstretched services) but at the same time cut down on inappropriate, avoidable referrals.

Mitchell (1985) described five models of a psychiatrist working with primary care staff in the context of adult community psychiatry:

1  co-ordinated home visits by GP and mental health worker
2  shift of psychiatric clinics to health centres or GP surgeries
3  visit to surgeries to see selected patients
4  group discussions with primary care staff
5  conjoint consultations.

All five models or a judicious mix of any number of them can be applied in day-to-day practice in the context of CAMHS. The experiences of both authors show that it is quite hard to start this anew; however, the rewards of going out and consulting with primary care staff are well worth it if a service gets established. A child psychiatrist can keep one session for consultation to primary care staff.

This session could be used for group consultation in a primary care setting, e.g. with health visitors, school nurses and social workers, with the consultant being available at a set time and letting people know by telephone as well as in writing. The consultant can also spend some time seeing one or two patients there who find it difficult to travel long distances to the clinic. It may also be useful to arrange a couple of multidisciplinary presentations to explain the referrals policy and ways in which primary care staff, including GPs, can screen for psychiatric disorders among children and adolescents. In the current climate, it is essential to identify local primary care trust (PCT) leads for mental health, particularly CAMH. GPs do appreciate a consultant who is available at the end of a telephone line for consultation and advice. Due to the diverse nature of their services, they also need to be reminded of the way local CAMHS prioritise and process their referrals.

## Paediatric consultation–liaison

Melvin Lewis (Lewis and Leebens 1996) has described various models of consultation derived in the American context, the names of which are self-explanatory:

- anticipatory model
- case-finding model
- education and training model
- emergency response model
- continuing and collaborative care model.

The authors of this chapter work in a service that uses all five models depending on the situation. Knowledge of these models and tailoring them to different consultation requests is an essential part of CAMHS work these days. In general, urgent requests for consultation come from hospital-based paediatricians and the nature of these is quite different from those coming from community paediatricians. There is considerable evidence that physical disorders and psychiatric disturbances in children and adolescents have a clear association in excess of what could be due to chance (Shugart 1991; Steiner *et al.* 1993). Authors have tried to give an account of various consultation requests that are processed in their service and how one can practically deal with them.

Requests for consultation may come from a consultant paediatrician or a junior doctor in paediatrics, nursing staff on the ward or sometimes teachers and play specialists working there. The requests usually fall into one of the following categories:

1 *Emergencies on the ward.* These can vary from a child admitted because of attempted suicide to a child showing severe emotional distress, or non-compliance with essential treatment, or severe behavioural disturbance, admitted for physical disorder. It is useful to anticipate these situations and have a duty rota of mental health professionals. In the service that the authors work in, there is first an on-call rota for attempted suicide (usually overdoses) operated by most of the mental health professionals in the service across geographical teams and a second on-call rota consisting of consultant child and adolescent psychiatrists. All referrals are filtered through the paediatric consultant responsible for the child.

It is not uncommon to come across a very disturbed young person on the paediatric wards, mainly due to an adjustment disorder to an unsafe or traumatising family situation rather than due to a primary psychiatric disorder. In our service we developed an integrated care pathway which incorporates joint working with social care and health. This evolved out of a series of consultations with senior social care and health staff members and specialist CAMHS members. It is still quite difficult to provide a seamless and comprehensive service for these very needy young people but at least there is an increasing awareness and acceptance of this problem.

2 *Requests for consultation for unexplained physical symptoms.* It is useful to have a close working relationship with paediatricians, making it more likely that a request will come in early before a long list of often exhaustive investigation has been completed. Paediatricians often refer a case to a child psychiatrist as a last resort or when they are unable to find a physical cause for the patient's difficulties. A close working relationship ensures that they include the child psychiatrists as a matter of routine for cases that they feel have a psychiatric component.

3 *Children with chronic physical disorders* such as asthma, diabetes mellitus, ulcerative mellitus or cystic fibrosis need considerable support for

psychological distress. Although some hospitals are in the fortunate position of having specialist teams whose focus is psychological medicine (*see* Chapter 8), in many cases such work is undertaken by CAMHS, often as part of a paediatric liaison service.

4 *Children developing symptoms of psychiatric disorder following somatic illness.* A prolonged illness for head injury or major operations followed by persistent difficulties in adjusting back to normal life may also trigger a request for a consultation.

5 *Acute stress reactions or post-traumatic stress disorders (PTSD).* Increasingly, child psychiatrists or psychologists can provide consultation to such requests and also get involved with treatment quite early on after trauma, rather than after the symptoms have become complicated by secondary consequences.

## School consultation

Schools are increasingly being expected to provide for students' mental health needs, especially when they impact on their academic performance. This is due to a variety of reasons:

- The incidence rate of problems like self-harm, eating disorders and substance abuse, including alcohol, is increasing and these are presenting at a younger age than before.
- Many mental health problems are being recognised as an association of developmental disorders such as Aspergers' syndrome, dyslexia, dyspraxia and so on. There has been rapid progress in what we know about causation as well as management of these disorders.
- Parents tend to be more aware about these developments through increasing influence of the media, especially the internet. This awareness, combined with high expectations about how children should be managed by professionals, has outpaced resources available on the ground. The numbers of professionals and resources available to them have not grown as fast as expectations and knowledge have in the last two to three decades.

In view of this climate, it is very important that CAMHS staff develop their skills of collaborating in a consultation exercise with schools. Every school is a complex social institution with its own rules, written and unwritten, as well as style and atmosphere. It is usually important to learn about the schools that are going to be offered consultation before starting the actual consultation exercise. Bostic and Rauch (1999) have described the three Rs of school consultation, which relate to 'relationships', 'recognition' and 'responses'. Although the authors describe consultation in the North American context, these are nevertheless valuable in informing clinical practice in the United Kingdom and the original article is worth reading. The three Rs are described in Box 7.2.

A senior nurse therapist runs a school consultation-cum-drop-in clinic in one of the geographical teams where the authors work. He combines consultation to staff (teachers and the school nurse) with occasional brief assessment followed by advice to staff. He is supported in this venture by his supervisor as well as the child psychiatrist in the team.

**Box 7.2 The three Rs**

1 **Relationships** – consultants should keep the long-term aim of strengthening the relationships of professionals dealing with the child in the school setting. This can be achieved by developing a professional, trusting and respectful relationship with the staff in the first instance. Often, containing staff anxiety or parental anxiety or facilitating the parent–staff relationship is a crucial outcome of consultation.

2 **Recognition** – recognising the systemic aspects of a unidimensional problem brought for consultation is an acquired complex skill. This includes recognising motivations of the child, staff, parents and resistances that have already been built into the system. This helps in finding ways of introducing systemic interventions aimed at realigning the dynamic forces between the child, parents and staff. Recognising defences used by parents or staff that lead to unrealistic expectations from the child is crucial when suggesting the interventions that are likely to give the child a chance to reach realistic goals.

3 **Responses** – facilitating helpful responses from staff to the child presenting with problems can be an outcome of a particular consultation or even an overall change in ethos as staff learn new skills which help contain their anxiety and arm them with strategies to deal with emotional or behavioural problems.

Case study 7.2

The parents of an 11-year-old child were very anxious about how he would adjust to transition from primary to secondary school. School staff perceived this as undermining of their authority and ability to deal with children with special needs. The nurse therapist could identify that the child had a mild degree of social communication disorder and had always needed extra support and time to adjust to any change. This understanding helped him facilitate negotiation between the school and parents and mobilise additional support for the child from the Local Education Authority during consultation to the school staff.

## Medico-legal settings

Mental health problems, including psychosis, suicidal depression and other serious diagnosable disorders, are quite common in vulnerable populations such as looked-after children and young offender institutions and prisons (Maden *et al.* 1995; *see also* Chapters 9 and 10). Social workers, probation officers or staff working in child care homes, and police officers dealing with juvenile offenders or child protection, can benefit from regular consultations with mental health professionals working in local CAMHS. Both authors are only too aware of how stretched core CAMHS are due to chronic underfunding and this has to be addressed first before undertaking this role. However, mental health professionals may use opportunities provided by consultation to create a common language across all agencies dealing with children and adolescents and more specifically their mental health. It is hoped that in the near future the National Service Framework for children's services will provide a clear framework and practical guidelines about this aspect of service provision.

Increasingly, mental health professionals are being called upon to offer consultation to staff working in medico-legal settings and this is becoming an essential part of a child psychiatrist's job. It is important for the professional undertaking such work to undergo regular training in the legal aspects of child mental health.

Whenever a request for consultation is made, the consultant can use a check-list of questions to gather essential information for quality consultation (*see* Box 7.3). This list is of course neither exhaustive nor universally applicable. It may be useful for professionals offering consultation to others to devise their own check-list, which can be updated from time to time.

## Consent and confidentiality

Children and adolescents are becoming aware of their rights from quite a young age and it is not uncommon to come across children wanting help without their parents' knowledge. It is the duty of the professional to make a judgement based on weighing the pros and cons of agreeing or disagreeing to a child's request. What action will be in the best interest of the child now and over the long term should be the guiding ethical principle above all legislative provisions. In general, it is unwise to offer absolute, unconditional confidentiality to children and young people, and for that matter, anyone. It is useful to clarify at the outset that, barring exceptional situations where there is concern for the well-being of the

---

**Box 7.3  Consultation check-list**

1   What is the role of the professional requesting consultation in relation to the child?
2   How old is the child and who has parental responsibility for him?
3   What is the specific question that the consultee wants answered through consultation?
4   Is the child under any legal orders under the Children's Act or Criminal Justice Act?
5   Does the consultee want a written report to produce in a court of law?
6   Is the consultation request about risk assessment, clinical formulation, information seeking or a mixture of all these elements? If it is the latter, can one unpick them?
7   What legal framework is relevant in the presenting situation (Mental Health Act 1983; Children Act 1989; Criminal Justice Act 1982; Family Law Act 1996; Adoption Act 1976)?

patient or another person on account of possible actions of the patient, everything said by the patient during the session will be kept confidential.

---

**Case study 7.3**

A GP requested consultation about a 12-year-old girl who attended surgery along with a female church worker. The girl wanted to access counselling as she was feeling depressed. However, she did not want her mother to know anything about her attendance at the surgery or any further treatment. She had also been cutting herself and presented as mostly uncommunicative with poor eye contact. The GP was concerned that if she overrode the patient's right to confidentiality on account of her concerns about risk to the girl's life, she may alienate her. During consultation it was suggested that the GP saw the girl again to ascertain the reasons behind her request for confidentiality from her parents. An offer of a joint consultation was made in order to make a judgement about whether the girl's competence to consent to treatment, irrespective of her age in this particular case, may override concerns regarding her protection as a child. The outcome of the joint consultation was that the GP decided to continue to see the girl regularly to establish and maintain rapport in addition to arranging counselling for her. This was arranged with absolute confidentiality via a voluntary agency. She was also given the option of seeking consultation or joint assessment as and when she felt it appropriate in the future.

---

This case example illustrates the principle used in the Gillick case (Gillick vs West Norfolk Wisbech Health Authority 1985) judgement in relation to offering help when applied to a mental health problem in a child. While deciding about a child's request for treatment in confidence from parents, the following points are relevant:

- The consequences of receiving or not receiving the treatment and whether the child is in a position to be able to trust the professional involved is a primary consideration. The child's capacity to understand the nature of the treatment may take precedence over parental powers and the child's chronological age. This can be overridden if necessary (e.g. in life-threatening situations such as anorexia nervosa). While this should be a useful provision in life-threatening situations, it may be ethically sounder to advise assessment under the Mental Health Act or to apply to the court to make a decision regarding treatment if the adolescent continues to refuse treatment over the long term.
- Parental powers dwindle as the child matures and they are mainly for protection of the child.
- The professional has also to think of possible adverse consequences of overriding the child's confidentiality against ensuring safety of the child by doing so.

The mental health professional should never lose sight of the fact that they are an expert in child mental health and not in the law, social work or police work. They should not be shy in asking for advice in legal matters unfamiliar to them but familiar to the consultee or an appropriate colleague. This will reduce anxiety that can come from entering uncharted territory. They should try to explore recent changes in the child's behaviour, the level of coping in context of their developmental level and how this correlates with the child's life history. They should not hesitate to seek advice through further expert assessments or psychometric tests, if these seem necessary in helping them to gain a full picture.

---

**Case study 7.4**

One CID officer requested consultation about a five-year-old girl who had witnessed her mother's murder. A specially trained child protection police worker had interviewed her. A couple of adult relatives had been referred to Victim Support but the officer wanted advice on what was best for the girl. On enquiry, it became clear that a large supportive network of her aunts and uncles was looking after her. She was living with an aunt that she had always been close to and had a cousin of similar age to play with. She appeared to be coping well at school and her sleep, appetite and mood appeared normal according to the officer's report. The officer was reassured that stability and containment and nurturing, caring of the girl by people that she was closely attached to, was the first priority. A referral was also made to the local CAMHS team to consider assessment of the girl with priority.

---

## Summary and conclusions

Consultation is a collaborative exercise between professionals where one of them offers their professional expertise to others in such a way as to facilitate thinking and problem solving. This role can be reversed among professionals depending on different areas of expertise. It is an important professional activity and cannot just be added on to other clinical work in spare time. Professionals should value it and assign ample time to practise it systematically. A record of consultations requested and offered is an essential aspect, which can easily be forgotten during a busy work schedule.

The same basic process of consultation can be modified to suit various settings, such as schools, paediatric wards, social care and health settings, and the medico-legal field. Apart from having a sound knowledge base, a consultant is helped by acquiring an experiential understanding of group processes, organisational dynamics and cultures.

A few dos and don'ts should be considered before embarking on consultation. Like most skilled activities, practice and experience over time combined with self-reflection may improve the quality of consultation.

## Acknowledgements

The authors would like to thank Mary Battison for word-processing, Suhrud Banhatti for help with the figure and Ruchi Banhatti for help with formatting.

# References

Bostic JQ and Rauch PK (1999) The three Rs of school consultation. *Journal of the American Academy of Child and Adolescent Psychiatry.* **38** (3): 339–41.

Gillick vs West Norfolk and Wisbech Health Authority and the Department of Health (1985) *Weekly Law Reports.* **3**: 830.

Kramer T and Garralda ME (1998) Psychiatric disorders in adolescents in primary care. *British Journal of Psychiatry.* **173**: 508–13.

Kramer T and Garralda ME (2000) Child and adolescent mental health problems in primary care. *Advances in Psychiatric Treatment.* **6**: 287–94.

Lewis M and Leebens PK (1996) The consultation process in child and adolescent psychiatric consultation–liaison in paediatrics. In: Lewis M (ed.) *Child and Adolescent Psychiatry: a comprehensive textbook* (2e), pp. 935–9. Williams and Wilkins, Baltimore, MD.

Maden A, Taylor CJA, Brooke D *et al.* (1995) *Mental Disorder in Remand Prisoners.* Home Office Research and Statistics Directorate Information Section, London.

Mitchell ARK (1985) Psychiatrists in primary health care settings. *British Journal of Psychiatry.* **147**: 371–9.

NHS Health Advisory Service (1995) *Child and Adolescent Mental Health Services: together we stand.* HMSO, London.

Shugart MA (1991) Child psychiatry consultations to paediatric inpatients: a literature review. *General Hospital Psychiatry.* **13**: 325–36.

Steiner H, Fritz GK, Mrazek D *et al.* (1993) Paediatric and psychiatric co-morbidity. Part I: The future of consultation–liaison psychiatry. *Psychosomatics.* **34** (2): 107–11.

# Chapter 8

# Consultation in paediatric psychology

*Mandy Bryon and Daniela Hearst*

## Introduction

The rapid advances in biomedical technology over the last 30 years have influenced fundamental changes in paediatric service delivery. The narrow pathology-based prescriptive model of care has yielded to a more holistic approach that emphasises the psychosocial factors and lifestyle that may enhance or compromise health and normal development. The child is no longer viewed in terms of isolated symptomatology but in the context of the family and wider community. The demand on paediatricians is not only to be more psychologically aware but also to work collaboratively with psychosocial colleagues, as part of a multidisciplinary team (Bingley *et al.* 1980; Klein 1985; Menahem 1987; Graham 1994).

Any number of mental health practitioners may, of course, be involved with children who have physical health problems and who have concurrent mental health needs (*see* Chapter 8). However, paediatric clinical psychologists have developed a unique focus and specialisation in child health and health-related psychological issues: this focus is distinct and complementary to that of the mental health team, as will be seen as the chapter unfolds. Most paediatric psychologists are integrated into the hospital paediatric team. Aside from their own clinical practice, their work involves enhancing others' psychological under-standing of children with health problems and ensuring that the psychosocial perspective is not lost. Trained clinical psychologists working in the paediatric setting fulfil a number of roles, including that of clinician, educator, trainer, researcher and consultant. The scarcity of paediatric psychologists, coupled with their core remit to support and develop psychological understanding and skills in others, has meant that consultation is often well developed in paediatric settings and is, indeed, the 'backbone' of many services.

This chapter focuses on indirect consultation with health professionals in which consultation is defined as a process of joint enquiry and exploration – an advice or help-giving relationship between consultee and consultant. In essence, con-sultation involves working with other people's perspectives, assumptions and expertise to address the needs of the child and family, consultee and medical teams as well as the broader social context of the problem (Steinberg 1989; Hamlett and Stabler 1995). As Drotar (1995) says, consultation '. . . aims to deliver an extraordinary product – a practical intervention plan that addresses the complexity of a problem quickly.'

Specific aims of consultation are to advocate for the child and family, clarify questions, reduce anxiety about the issue (and the consultant!), enhance understanding, add a different perspective, empower the consultee, foster confidence, educate, increase problem-solving skills and strengthen relationships – professional and between professionals and families. Consultation can occur in a variety of ways, from 'can I just ask a quick question?' in the corridor to regular psychosocial meetings, staff teaching and support, via specific protocols and increasingly by telephone.

This chapter considers some of the core aspects of the consultation process in paediatrics using case examples to illustrate a number of different consultation situations. Before doing so, however, it is important to provide the reader with some summary information about the background and context of paediatric psychology, as well as the theoretical model that underpins this work: all of these things shape the consultation process.

## Paediatric psychology: the context

Paediatric psychologists have needed to adapt well-established models of service delivery advocated within a mental health setting to that of the paediatric hospital. As a potential member of a multidisciplinary team, it may be the psychologist's role to establish that team, in which they may well be the only mental health professional, in contrast to traditional child and adolescent mental health teams. The paediatric medical staff may not have experience of identifying and referring psychological issues. A significant part of the psychologist's role will therefore be educative. Effective psychological service provision in a paediatric team will include a range of differing models of delivery, including psychosocial ward rounds, integrated medical/psychological outpatient clinics, ward and bed-side consultation, and liaison both internally and externally.

The essence of a successful consultation–liaison service is the close, collaborative working between medical and psychological disciplines (Sollner *et al.* 2002). This goes beyond a simple model of consultation in which professionals work independently on the same case and requires the psychologist to be an integrated member of the paediatric team, participating in case discussions, ward rounds and conferences as well as education programmes.

Paediatric psychology is increasingly being purchased at secondary (district general hospital) level for general paediatric wards and clinics. Increasingly, this is tending to include dedicated time for specialist clinics of more common chronic illnesses such as asthma and diabetes. It remains the case, however, that the majority of paediatric psychology is provided at tertiary level in specialist paediatric centres. Here, any psychological intervention may be more time-limited or logistically difficult, requiring close liaison and shared care plans with other levels of National Health Service (NHS) care, e.g. local hospitals and community services. This has amplified the need for alternative kinds of psychological service delivery, including indirect psychological consultation.

## Theoretical model

Central to and underpinning consultation is the theoretical model of paediatric psychology. In contrast to the mental health services, paediatric psychology focuses on normal developmental trajectories with the emphasis on individual and family strengths and resiliencies that reduce the trauma of illness and disability and enable maximal adaptation. The picture is one of a normal child and family living with and adapting to abnormal circumstances (Eiser 1994). Moving away from what could be described as a narrow, prescriptive medical model, the role of the paediatric psychologist is more often proactive and preventative, rather than reactive to pre-diagnosed clinical 'pathology'. Consultation highlights this collaborative, non-pathologising way of working, through a reframing of 'symptoms' as questions and hypotheses that reflect normal developmental challenges and reinforce appropriate emotional responses.

## Definition and aims of consultation

Paediatricians and health professionals are increasingly adopting a patient-centred and more holistic approach to medicine (Lewin *et al.* 2003). Within routine medical consultations, the paediatrician will come across what are perceived as difficult situations at the outer limits of their medical skills and where more psychosocial knowledge is appropriate (Hewson *et al.* 1999; Cooper and Hewson 2002). At this point a consultation–liaison psychology service can be utilised and there are a range of ways that consultation can occur, ranging from 'direct' face-to-face consultation to team discussion, as shown in Box 8.1.

---

**Box 8.1 Different types of paediatric consultation**

- Face-to-face patient consultation with the psychologist
- Consultation to health professional (indirect)
- Psychosocial perspective added to case discussion
- Team discussion to teach psychosocial concepts

---

## Influencing factors

As with any system of psychological intervention, the success or failure of indirect consultation does not solely depend on the expertise and experience of the consultant but is strongly influenced by the context, structures and systems in which the consultation is delivered. Medical hierarchies, training, assumptions and styles all influence the process.

Indirect consultation can have long-lasting and wide-ranging effects beyond the outcome of an individual case or issue. It can help create or enhance relationships and communication between professionals of different disciplines with the knock-on effect of improving future referral questions. It fosters increased psychological understanding in the paediatric team, which enhances practice and longer-term planning, thereby improving care for a larger population of children.

Conversely, consultation has its pitfalls: it is time-consuming and demanding and expectations may not be made explicit. The doctor or nurse, as consultee, may not want to be empowered to solve the problem themselves but expect the consultant to provide an instant, 'quick fix' solution to a complex problem. Attempts made to reframe problems can be strongly resisted!

Such impediments to psychosocial consultation in the paediatric setting stem from differences in the training and theoretical stance of medical and psychosocial professionals. There is a traditional and rigid model of medical provision that pervades the health service. This establishes and maintains a strict hierarchy of authority that in many cases precludes consultation and collaboration with other disciplines. There is an imbalance of power in favour of medical consultants and the hospital system that puts other professionals and patients at the receiving end of a prescriptive model. Efforts to challenge the traditional medical model have been increasingly successful and good advice on how to establish psychosocial consultation–liaison services is now available. Kush and Campo (1998) argue that to effectively deliver a medical service, a knowledge of the psychosocial needs of the patient is essential as well as understanding when the medical diagnosis gives way to more appropriate psychological management. Thus, they describe the requirement of psychosocial liaison as well as the importance of the inclusion of psychology in medical training.

The patient-centred or needs-led approach to health provision is fast becoming the best practice model of service delivery. This follows logically from the recommendations of several recent NHS inquiries into events where parent consultation and inclusion in decisions about their children's care was not part of routine clinical practice. The establishment of patient forums and patient membership of ethics committees (Smyth 2001) in order that they have influence on health service provision and research is a clear indication that large philosophical shifts in the delivery of medicine are occurring at strategic levels (Department of Health, 2003).

## Process of consultation

It is often difficult as a clinician to notice when the process of consultation starts; within a busy paediatric service opinions are frequently and quickly sought. It is worthwhile, therefore, delineating the process of consultation so that more consideration may be given to this invaluable skill. The clinician offering psychological consultation will need to:

- *consider the time-scale:* consultation delivery needs to be appropriate to the setting and busy schedules. The consultant must be readily available and able to ensure a fast response time when, for example, an imminent procedure is scheduled or the child is to be discharged
- *look beyond the surface request:* consultation triggered by family distress, non-adherence to treatment in the child or angry parents may mask underlying issues, e.g. professional conflicts within medical/nursing team or need for staff support
- *negotiate responsibilities for actions and interventions:* an explicit agreement must be reached on who will take what action, based on the outcome of the consultation. The consultee is likely to want a quick solution and may hope or just assume that the psychologist will immediately take on the case
- *negotiate realistic expectations and goals:* assumptions on both sides based on different professional trainings are all too easily made about what can or

should be done and in what time-scale. The consultant must remain mindful of the delicate balance between fostering the consultee's confidence to gain new experience and psychological skills and pushing too far beyond their boundaries of professional competence

- *translate* psychological knowledge into a jargon-free practical form
- *communicate* clearly with responses that are prompt, brief, factual and highly specific, as necessary
- be a *'humble expert'* (Drotar 1995): the consultant must take care not to dominate the interaction and be a psychological 'know-all' but be able to share their experience and knowledge without undermining the skills or effectiveness of the consultee
- take a *non-competitive approach* and cultivate a truly collaborative, multi-disciplinary ethos
- *acknowledge differing professional language, narratives and culture:* e.g. the expression of distress or downright misery in sick children can readily be pathologised into a diagnosis of depression. Similarly, ward staff can be quick to label parental adjustment to and coping with their child's illness as inappropriate, based on their judgements of what level of emotion is 'normal' for fathers and mothers to display: too few tears becomes 'denial', too many, 'depression'
- *interpret and collate observations* – often incomplete – and 'facts' collected by others. The consultant may wish to help the consultee to reframe a prescriptive psychiatric-type diagnosis as a description of behaviour and development that emphasises functional adaptation and competencies, as well as 'deficits' and vulnerabilities in the face of adverse life events and constraints.

---

**Box 8.2 Important considerations in paediatric consultation**

- Time-scale: sometimes an immediate response is required
- Looking beyond the surface request
- Negotiating responsibilities for actions and interventions
- Negotiating realistic expectations and goals
- Translating 'expert' knowledge into jargon-free language
- Adopting a non-expert position
- Acknowledging different professional language, narratives and culture

The consultant's observations help to provide a bigger picture that generates alternative ideas about the problem.

---

In essence the consultation process should be:

- *collaborative* rather than expert
- *consultee retaining control* rather than the consultant
- *empowering* for the consultee rather than disempowering.

## The need for co-ordination

The establishment of psychosocial services in paediatric settings is often piece-meal, resulting in disjointed services that can affect the process of consultation. For example, some hospitals have separate departments of psychosocially trained professionals, such as psychologists, psychiatrists and social workers, all of whom may be consulted about the same case. Ward staff may 'fire off' referrals in the hope that one will be successful. This can often result in confusing consultations for the patient and the ward staff. A co-ordinated approach to psychosocial service provision is obviously more sensible and models of such multidisciplinary approaches demonstrate the advantages of a concise and unified approach, providing both a forum for informal consultation and teaching opportunities.

## Case studies

The following cases are offered as examples of indirect consultations to individuals, single and multiple professional groups with notes on aims, process and outcome.

---

**Case study 8.1 Providing a link between paediatric and adult services: consultation to the adult cystic fibrosis team**

With advances in medical care, many children with cystic fibrosis (CF) are now surviving past adolescence and into early adulthood; this necessitates children and their families leaving their paediatric medical team and moving to specialist respiratory services for adults located at other hospitals. Families and the medical team who have known each other for years can become very attached: it can be as hard for the medical team to 'give up' their patients as it is for families to move on to adult services. Transition from paediatric to adult services is a planned for, gradual and carefully managed process.

At the specialist children's hospital, the multidisciplinary CF team, which includes a consultant clinical psychologist, has worked together for many years. The team holds weekly psychosocial meetings at which any patient of concern is discussed.

Two years ago, one of the specialist nurses in CF left the children's hospital to take up a post in a different trust, working with adult CF patients. She discovered a distinct lack of a psychosocial perspective in her new team and found it extremely difficult to access advice or help on psychological issues. Increasingly concerned by her perceived inability to meet the psychological needs of her adult patients, the specialist nurse approached her ex-colleague, the clinical psychologist in the paediatric service, for help. After discussions with both her paediatric team and the adult CF service it was agreed that the psychologist would offer consultation to the adult team in a series of monthly meetings held at the adult hospital.

---

Regular consultation helped team members become more confident in their own abilities. As this happened, the focus of the consultation meetings shifted: instead of requesting direct advice on psychological interventions, the team worked with the consultant to formulate psychological issues using a developmental, normative framework and to devise management strategies.

The specialist nurse became more confident in her own skills in dealing with any psychological problems her patients presented; this confidence included her ability to recognise when she had reached the limits of her professional competence and needed to refer on for specialist services.

Within a year, discussion sessions extended to include issues that affected team functioning and future services planning. Most recently, the team decided they wanted a psychologist 'of their own' and in their business plan for new service developments included a proposal for dedicated psychology sessions.

## Comments

- As the consultant was an employee of a separate NHS trust, the boundaries of consultation needed to be clearly maintained. The consultant was not asked to see patients directly and the consultees remained the primary and sole care providers. Care was taken to protect patients' identity.
- The consultee group initially described their concerns about their patients in terms of symptoms or pathological behaviours. Over time, the consultant promoted the use of a non-pathologising, developmental framework, in which 'symptoms' could be reframed in terms of developmental challenges of chronic illness. Possible psychological interventions were placed in a context of family strengths, resiliencies and coping strategies. Reframing the psychological narrative allowed the team to develop a perspective that could be applied to all their patients.
- The process of consultation is as important as the content; over time trust grew, both between the consultee group and the consultant and among the team members. The consultant also became the team's facilitator, enabling team members to safely examine and strengthen their professional roles, relationships and ways of working together.
- The consultant offered expertise in a manner to foster and encourage the consultees' confidence and competence to deliver psychosocial care. Training and transferral skills do preclude the need for the services of an experienced psychologist. As the consultees developed their skills, these included an awareness of the boundaries of their competence, experience and training, so that they could identify patients and families who needed referral for more specialist help.
- Consultation can lead to new service developments which impact on a whole population of patients.

## Summary

---

**Consultation outcomes**

- Resolution of individual patient issues
- Team education and improved functioning
- Opportunity for service development, affecting wider client population

---

---

**Case study 8.2 Consultation to the anaesthetic department: unexpected developments**

Out of the blue, one of the consultant clinical psychologists received a request from the head of the paediatric anaesthetic department to speak at a departmental seminar on the subject of management of behavioural distress in children undergoing surgery. The invitation came as a surprise: whilst specialist psychologists offer services to the majority of medical/surgical specialties, there had been minimal interaction with the anaesthetists as a professional group.

The lecture was scheduled at 7.30 a.m. – a salutary experience for the psychologist – and covered incidence and developmental patterns of behavioural distress with age, predictors of pre- and peri-operative anxiety for child and family, and anxiety management strategies. It provoked animated discussion within the group, as both experienced and junior anaesthetists in training shared their most challenging cases. These tended to be children who unexpectedly became so distressed and agitated in the anaesthetic room that the surgical procedure had to be delayed or even cancelled, with the consequent disruption to the busy theatre schedule. The anaesthetists wanted to know how to restore calm and effectively enable a distraught child to undergo anaesthesia.

The psychologist acknowledged both the difficulty of the problem as well as her own lack of direct experience working with children in the anaesthetic room. She offered a range of possible management strategies based on proactive preventative work and agreed to spend a day with them in theatres to study the problem at first hand.

A ten-hour day of observation in theatres revealed the pressures and tensions on both children and staff; various suggestions to reduce peri-operative stress were proposed by the psychologist. This led not only to explorations of how best to manage children's distress but also to the development of a collaborative research proposal to attempt to identify those children whose high levels of anxiety and distress threatened anaesthetic induction. A further outcome of the process was the inclusion of the psychologist as a contributor to the training courses offered by the paediatric anaesthetists to non-specialist colleagues outside the hospital.

---

## Comments

- The anaesthetist consultees wanted an instant solution to the acute problem of resistance to anaesthesia. It would have been foolish, if not downright arrogant of the psychologist to suggest she held the key to the magic 'quick fix'. Instead the consultation concentrated on broadening the context of the problem, looking at the wider issue of identification and reduction of distress. It was important to acknowledge that often there is no immediate or obvious single solution.
- It was important to understand the context in which the anaesthetists' concerns arose – hence the day spent in theatres. This opportunity for direct observation served a dual purpose:
  - it maximised the usefulness and applicability of any suggestions to improve practice by helping the psychologist gain a broader understanding of the procedures involved and experiences of children and their parents at a time of high anxiety
  - it helped the psychologist to better appreciate the pressures on the anaesthetists to ensure smooth running of the surgical list.
- One opportunity often leads to many others: in this case the chance to improve patient care, offer training in psychological issues to wider professional groups and develop collaborative research and development projects.

## Summary

---

### Consultation outcomes

- Education to hospital staff and wider professional audiences
- Offering a psychological dimension to anaesthetic practice
- Longer-term collaborative work
- Modified clinical practice affecting a wide client group

---

### Case study 8.3 Helping others cope with trauma: telephone consultation

An urgent request for paediatric psychology services arrived, via a secretary, from the surgical intensive care unit of a neighbouring hospital specialising in adult neurological diseases. The psychologist called the unit and spoke to the staff nurse; the nurse asked if a paediatric psychologist could come to the unit the following evening to counsel the two young children of her patient. The patient was a 34-year-old woman, who had unexpectedly suffered a severe brain haemorrhage the previous weekend and, following emergency surgery, was unconscious and fully ventilated. She was now on the critical list and not expected to survive.

Her husband and children were in a state of shock and extreme distress; the children were due to visit their mother the following afternoon and the

*Continued*

nurse wanted a paediatric psychologist present in case they were over-whelmed by the appearance of their mother and the intensive care unit.

The nurse provided further details of the family and indicated her own distress at feeling out of her depth with the anxiety and distress of the family. The psychologist did not offer to visit the children; instead she spent extended time on the phone with the nurse exploring the children's possible beliefs and fears in the context of their developmental stages. On exploration, the nurse suggested various strategies to help the children during their visit and it became evident that she possessed more than adequate skills and competence to offer the children the appropriate support to help them deal with what was happening to their mother. Eventually, the nurse began to question whether a psychologist was needed at this stage. The psychologist agreed that it could be counter-productive to introduce an unfamiliar adult at an already stressful time. The nurse mentioned the children's father's request for advice and suitable materials to use with his children, should his wife die. The psychologist promised to make these available to the nurse, if needed, but also suggested that this might be looking too far into the future and that it would be important to maintain reasonable hope and concentrate on the short term. The psychologist arranged to speak to the nurse the next evening to see how the visit had gone.

Evidently the children had coped well; the nurse met the family outside the unit and reinforced the preparation the father had already given his children, in terms of answering their questions simply and honestly and explaining what the children could expect to see and hear. The children appeared reassured and curious, rather than upset, to see the machinery surrounding her. The nurse observed, with some surprise, that both children appeared much less distressed after their visit. Possible reasons for this were discussed. It was mutually agreed that the psychologist would not meet the children but that she would be available to consult with the nurse as required.

Two weeks later, a different nurse requested advice on another patient in the same unit and this was offered. Following this, the consultant intensivist in charge of the unit approached the psychologist to negotiate the possibility of establishing regular consultation sessions to all her staff.

## Comments

- The initial request is often for a direct intervention with a child and family – even when judged clinically inappropriate and logistically difficult. For example, in this case there was no formal agreement between the specialist hospitals to see each other's patients. The consultee may not see themselves in the role of consultee, but that of prospective referrer. Thus the consultant's apparent 'non-acceptance' of the referral may be interpreted as lack of co-operation. It is important for the consultant to spend enough time with the referrer, whether face to face or on the phone, so that the consultee feels their concerns have been properly discussed and an acceptable solution negotiated.

- It was important that the children's distress and anxiety were viewed in a normal developmental framework and not as symptoms of pathology needing therapy.
- The consultation reinforced the psychological knowledge and skills of the nurse, so that she felt competent to offer the appropriate support.
- Useful consultation can be offered even to unknown colleagues in a different medical setting.
- The consultant must learn to curb their curiosity and tolerate not knowing the outcome; indeed it may be proof of the success of the consultation when no more is heard and the consultant has evidently become redundant to the case.
- A successful consultation can lead to new opportunities to create new education/training programmes that have a wider audience and potentially affect a larger patient population.

## Summary

---

**Consultation outcomes**

- Increased confidence in consultee to manage the problem
- Appropriate care offered to family by a familiar professional
- Children's distress not pathologised but reframed in a developmental context
- Request for new consultation service and opportunity for continued liaison and collaboration between paediatric and adult services

---

**Case study 8.4 A bereavement on the renal unit: dealing with staff anxieties**

Psychologists offer an on-call emergency service to the hospital and cover each other over periods of absence, as well as providing an emergency service to those specialties without dedicated psychosocial staff. On-call rotas ensure a named psychologist is available each day.

The on-call psychologist received a phone call from the sister on the renal unit requesting that a child be seen for assessment. The eight-year-old girl was a day patient, attending for dialysis, and was causing concern to the nursing staff as she appeared extremely distressed and withdrawn following the death of a close friend in the intensive care unit. Members of the unit psychosocial team were on leave and not available; the sister thought the girl might need treatment for 'depression'.

Over the phone, the psychologist discussed the context of the child's behaviour, the recent events leading up to the friend's death, her family's responses and the wider network of social support available to the child. It emerged that the nursing staff were not concerned that the girl was at risk of self-harm, nor on detailed questioning was there any indication of clinical depression.

*Continued*

The ensuing discussion focused on the ways an eight-year-old might react and grieve for the loss of her friend, especially in a context of her own life-limiting illness. The ward sister, who knew the family well, thought she would discuss the situation with the parents and obtain their agreement for her to speak to their daughter about her friend's death and possible concerns about her own state of health. The sister also agreed that an 'emergency' psychological assessment was not indicated at this stage and, given the imminent return of members of the psychosocial team, could be deferred. The psychologist agreed to liaise with the psychosocial team and would meanwhile remain available to the sister and child if needed.

A call back to the ward two days later established that the girl was very sad but eager to speak to nursing staff about her worries and feelings. Staff concerns about her psychological state had diminished.

## Comments

- Anxiety about a possible clinical depression was acknowledged and contained. Symptoms were reframed and normalised in terms of developmentally appropriate distress.
- It was important to ensure attention was paid to the support network available to the child outside the hospital and involve the family as experts in helping to manage the problem.
- The consultee was enabled to propose and implement her own intervention with the consultant remaining available for proactive support.

## Summary

**Consultation outcomes**

- Grief facilitated, not pathologised
- Consultee's skills reinforced and promoted
- Specialist assessment rendered redundant

**Case study 8.5  Invasive procedures**

The on-call psychologist received a call from the day investigations unit (which does not have dedicated psychosocial input) for help with a three-year-old boy who required invasive procedures the next day, including a blood test. The child was observed to be restless, distractible and aggressive, hitting out indiscriminately, whenever a nurse entered the room. Staff felt that the boy's mother was inappropriately tolerant of her son's negative behaviour towards them.

The psychologist met with the ward's staff nurse, junior doctor, play therapist and the child's mother within two hours. The mother told staff of her own fear of needles and how she felt helpless in supporting her son through the necessary investigations.

The doctor went over the proposed schedule of tests and it was decided to proceed without the blood test; instead oral sedatives would be given so that a canula could be inserted. A plan was drawn up between ward staff and mother to agree exactly how, when and where the procedures would be conducted and the degree of choice available to the child during the medical tests. The blood test would be deferred to a later date which would allow the play therapist time to work with the child and mother on distraction techniques and other coping strategies, as an outpatient. It emerged that regular blood tests would be required but, if preferred by the mother, these could be undertaken at their local hospital. The psychologist agreed to remain available to the ward team for consultation until investigations were completed but also to try and arrange for local psychological help for the family, as necessary. The investigations took place the next day; the nurses noted both the child and his mother appeared calmer. There were two further consultations with the nurses and play therapist and the blood test was successfully obtained at an outpatient appointment two weeks later.

## Comments

- An important aspect of the consultation was the availability and speed of response from the consultant. In hospital settings, it is essential to set aside time on on-call days so that schedules can be rearranged as circumstances demand.
- The ward staff experienced the child's behaviour as challenging and his mother's as inconsistent. Including the mother in the 'problem-solving team' diffused a potentially adversarial situation, strengthened the mother's expertise and coping abilities, and facilitated the negotiation of a medical schedule that the boy could tolerate.
- Rare is the occasion of the instant solution to the problems frequently presented in specialist paediatric consultations. This consultation was unlikely to produce a 'magic' way of immediately procuring the child's adherence to aversive and invasive procedures. Instead the consultant facilitated a medically agreed change to the proposed schedule of investigations and the creation of 'breathing space' for the family in which there was the possibility of helping the child and mother cope with the longer-term challenge of repeated blood tests.

## Summary

---

**Consultation outcomes**

- Improved adherence to medical protocol in both the short and longer term
- Closer working relationships between ward staff
- Increased awareness of parental concerns

---

# Summary and implications for future practice and research

A survey of 89 psychologists working in child and paediatric settings in the USA concluded that future training should emphasise brief treatment techniques and consultation/liaison skills (Walker 1989). Clearly, the above case studies illustrate the value of indirect consultation in empowering other disciplines, more effective intervention by appropriate staff, development of further necessary services and the inclusion of the patient's wishes in consideration of treatment provision, amongst others.

The use of telephone consultation has been debated recently as a means of rapid response to patients, to increase efficiency and reduce time and costs of face-to-face contacts. The reports have found varying benefits with the indication that telephone consultation in primary care is superficially cost-effective as the majority of patients contacted by telephone were 1.5 times more likely to turn up for a face-to-face follow-up than those who presented to the surgery for consultation (McKinstry 2002).

Telephone consultation in chronic illness management was, however, reported to be an essential part of service delivery. It is suggested that illnesses requiring complex daily management can be effectively managed by quick consultations to the appropriate member of a multidisciplinary team (Taccetti 2002). A large part of clinical psychology consultation in the paediatric setting is necessarily carried out by telephone. Adequate multidisciplinary care requires liaison to other agencies or colleagues in the patient's local community as well as continued contact, perhaps remotely, with the child and family. Telephone consultation in paediatric psychology is widely used but has not been the subject of good evaluation. This is certainly an area where clear formulation of types of telephone usage and investigation of efficacy would be useful.

In summary, to offer effective consultation, the psychologist needs to make use of the information given and negotiate responsibilities between themselves and those receiving the guidance that may then be directly applied to the patient. It is important that the psychologist feels comfortable that the consultee is capable of applying psychosocial strategies and not all cases will be amenable to indirect consultation.

Consultation is not a means of offering a less time-consuming service. The consultant needs to show commitment to the process by being available and taking over the intervention if it becomes indicated. It is essential that the consultant shows tolerance of the differences between disciplines in training, boundaries and theoretical understanding, and is cognisant of the context, setting and system in which the consultee works. Consultation skills are still, by and large, acquired through experience rather than formal teaching and how these skills are best developed is an important issue for post-qualification training and continued professional development.

Consultation by psychologists in the paediatric setting is valued and frequently requested. The potential benefits are for improved clinical outcome in the child and increased collaboration between disciplines that can lead to more teaching, training and better-designed services. Research is indicated to enhance collaborative practice and to evaluate indirect consultation, not just in clinical efficacy but also in terms of cost-effectiveness.

# References

Bingley L, Leonard J, Hensman S *et al.* (1980) Comprehensive management of children on a paediatric ward: a family approach. *Archives of Diseases in Childhood.* **55**: 555–61.

Cooper CP and Hewson PH (2002) The most difficult clinical situations: a survey of Victorian general practitioners. *Journal of Paediatrics and Child Health.* **38**: 455–8.

Department of Health (2003) *National Service Framework for Children.* HMSO, London.

Drotar D (1995) *Consulting with Paediatricians: psychological perspectives.* Plenum Press, New York.

Eiser C (1994) Making sense of chronic disease: the eleventh Jack Tizard memorial lecture. *Journal of Child Psychology and Psychiatry.* **33** (8): 1373–89.

Graham PJ (1994) Paediatrics and child psychiatry: past, present and future. *Acta Paediatrica.* **83**: 880–3.

Hamlett KW and Stabler B (1995) The developmental progress of pediatric psychology consultation. In: Roberts MC (ed.) *Handbook of Pediatric Psychology* (2e), pp. 39–54. Guilford Press, New York.

Hewson PH, Anderson PK, Dinning AH *et al.* (1999) A 12-month profile of community paediatric consultations in the Barwon region. *Journal of Paediatrics and Child Health.* **35**: 16–22.

Klein M (1985) Canadian departments of pediatrics and family medicine: in need of family therapy? *Canadian Medical Association Journal.* **15**: 629–33.

Kush SA and Campo JV (1998) Consultation and liaison in the paediatric setting. In: Ammerman RT and Campo JV (eds) *Handbook of Pediatric Psychology and Psychiatry, Vol. 1,* pp. 23–40. Allyn and Bacon, Needham Heights, MA.

Lewin SA, Skea ZC, Entwistle V *et al.* (2003) *Interventions for Providers to Promote a Patient-centred Approach in Clinical Consultations* (Cochrane review). The Cochrane Library, Issue 1. Update Software Ltd. www.update-software.com

McKinstry BH (2002) Telephone consultations may not save time. *British Medical Journal.* **325**: 1242.

Menahem S (1987) The contribution of the paediatrician and psychiatrist to the management of the child, adolescent and his family: a paediatrician's viewpoint. *Australian Paediatric Journal.* **23**: 235–9.

Smyth RL (2001) Research with children. *British Medical Journal.* **322**: 1377–8.

Sollner W, Stix P, Stein B *et al.* (2002) Quality criteria for psychosomatic consultation–liaison service. *Wein Med Wochenschr.* **152**: 528–34.

Steinberg D (1989) *Interprofessional Consultation: innovations and imagination in working relationships.* Blackwell Scientific, Oxford.

Taccetti G (2002) Telephone consultations in chronic diseases: an experience in cystic fibrosis. *British Medical Journal.* **324**: 1230–1.

Walker EC (1989) The future of pediatric psychology. *Pediatric Psychology.* **13**: 465–77.

# Chapter 9

# Consulting with youth offending teams

*Scott Sinclair and Kevin Epps*

## Introduction

This chapter is concerned with the development of consultancy approaches to working with youth offending teams (YOTs). The first part of the chapter provides the reader with background information on the development, structure and role of YOTs. Some of the issues faced by YOT practitioners will be discussed, with a particular emphasis on considering the mental health needs of young offenders. The chapter then moves on to explore some of the reasons why external consultancy services have been sought by YOT managers and practitioners. It also explores possible approaches to consultancy and raises issues that need to be considered before embarking on this type of work. The final part of the chapter provides an outline of a consultancy service developed in South Staffordshire, looking at the development of the service and noting some of the lessons learned along the way.

## Youth offending teams

In England and Wales, YOTs operating under the auspices of the Youth Justice Board (YJB) were established as a statutory requirement under Section 39 of the Crime and Disorder Act 1998. This Act set out a number of youth justice reforms following a highly critical report on youth justice by the Audit Commission, entitled 'Misspent Youth'. One of the requirements of this Act was that each local authority with responsibility for education and social services was to establish a multi-agency YOT with representation from the police, probation service, social services, health service and education. The principal aim of these teams is to prevent offending by children and young people.

Young people aged 10–17 years who offend or who are accused of offending can be referred to YOTs by any agency providing a children's service – most referrals come from the police or Courts. In England and Wales the age of criminal responsibility is ten years. (The National Probation Service and Adult Forensic Services deal with offenders aged 17 years and above.) All referrals to YOTs are assessed using a standardised assessment tool, the ASSET, which sets out critical factors associated with offending. This is completed by the YOT practitioner assigned to oversee the young person's progress (the 'case manager'). The information is collated from interviews with the young person and others involved with their care. The ASSET guides the case manager in ensuring that services and interventions are put in place to help reduce the risk of the young person reoffending. Sharing of information between agencies is seen as critical to the effectiveness and reliability of these assessments. The ASSET also aims to specify the likely risks that the young person presents to others.

From the point of a young person's arrest through to the completion of their sentence, YOTs deliver a wide range of services. They:

- provide assessments and reports for the Courts
- directly supervise young offenders (e.g. bail supervision, community sentences, the use of 'tagging')
- adopt 'restorative justice' approaches to give victims and communities a greater sense of being treated fairly
- help parents to become more effective in supervising their children (if necessary by means of a Parenting Order)
- work with the young person's school to improve school attendance and educational performance
- help the young person obtain training placements and employment
- supervise leisure activities
- provide short-term counselling or group work with young offenders to initiate behavioural changes
- support those serving custodial sentences (e.g. post-release care planning)
- carry out prevention work with the most at-risk young people in high crime areas
- make use of police final warnings as an intervention with young people and their families to prevent them drifting into further criminal activity.

## Youth crime

The true extent of offending among young people is unknown. It is accepted that a significant proportion of crime (defined here as an act that is capable of being followed by criminal proceedings) goes unreported (the so-called 'dark-figure'). Official estimates (based on a combination of sources, including the British Crime Survey, police-reported crime figures, Home Office statistics on cautions and convictions, and the YJB annual survey of youth crime) are therefore considered to be the 'tip of the iceberg'. However, it is also the case that most offences committed by young people are relatively minor, including acts such as fare-dodging on public transport and minor acts of vandalism. Offending is also more common in boys and tends to be a passing phase, reaching a peak around the age of 16 years and declining thereafter. In fact, despite the widespread prevalence of offending among young people, very few end up in conflict with the police and juvenile justice system. Of these, an even smaller proportion receive a criminal conviction and can rightly be termed 'young offenders' (Rutter et al. 1998).

Statistics collated during 2001 by the YJB, based on young people referred to YOTs, give some idea of who is likely to be offending within the 10–17 year range (Youth Justice Board 2002). Only 8% were aged between ten and 12 years whilst 70% fell into the 15–17 year range. Over half the young people were aged between 16 and 17 and only 16% were female. Those not regularly in school were found to commit three to four times more crime than those in school and their offences tended to be more serious. Many of the young people were found to be living in single-parent families, with only 30% living with both parents. Low educational attainment was also found to be common, with 41% regularly truanting from school and 60% assessed as having special educational needs. Many of the young people seen by YOT practitioners are also involved in regular substance misuse, with more than 50% using cannabis and in excess of 75% smoking and drinking alcohol. With respect to types of offending behaviour, YJB statistics for 2001 indicate that theft and handling is the most common offence (almost 60 000 young people), followed by violence against the person, motoring offences and criminal damage.

## Meeting the health needs of young offenders

Historically, the health of young offenders has received little attention. The primary focus of most interventions has been the reduction of offending, with minimal involvement from health services. The requirement of YOTs to include a health practitioner is therefore one of the more challenging innovations. Traditionally, most health workers have had little direct contact with young offenders, many of whom have become socially excluded and tend to bypass traditional referral routes via educational or primary care services. Some young offenders, for example, are not registered with a general practitioner.

The role of the health worker has certainly given rise to some uncertainty and confusion. This has arisen partly because YOT health workers have been recruited from diverse professional backgrounds. Many YOTs employ health workers with a general nursing background, often with experience of working in community settings. Others, however, employ nurses with a background in mental health, some with particular training and expertise in substance misuse, whilst others employ the services of clinical psychologists. In theory, the role of the health worker is to provide a focal point for health assessments and interventions, drawing on external health resources as necessary and using established links and professional contacts. However, the professional training and background of the health worker inevitably influences the overall character and development of the YOT, with some teams placing greater emphasis on physical health issues (e.g. medical history, physical examination, dental health), whilst other teams have been more concerned with the young person's mental health, spending more time assessing and reporting on mental health issues. These differences in professional orientation and emphasis inevitably lead to different patterns of referral to local external health providers, with some YOTs placing greater pressure on local child and adolescent mental health services (CAMHS).

There is, in fact, a great deal of confusion about the prevalence of mental health problems in the population of young people seen by YOTs. This confusion impinges on the work of all YOT workers, particularly the health workers, and also on external professionals including those who consult with YOTs. One of the challenges faced by all mental health workers at the present time is the task of explaining to a wider audience what exactly is meant by the terms 'mental health' and 'mental illness'. Historically, there has been a lack of communication and consensus about these core concepts between, and within, the various academic and professional disciplines represented in mental health services, including psychiatry, psychology and nursing. Different conceptual and definitional frameworks have been used to describe and understand mental health, informed by various ideologies and theories. The resulting confusion is, unfortunately, now causing difficulty in dealings with professional groups with little mental health training or experience. Where they seek clarity and understanding they find none. Experience also suggests that the term 'mental health' is unpopular with young people. The word 'mental' is often used in a derogatory manner (i.e. 'you're mental') and does not endear young people to services provided by 'mental health' professionals.

## The mental health of young offenders

According to research, increasing numbers of young people are being identified as having mental health problems and it has been estimated that up to one in five young people have psychological problems severe enough to require professional support (Rutter and Smith 1995). While there is debate about the full extent of mental health problems among young offenders, research evidence is consistent in showing that young people involved with the criminal justice system have elevated rates of mental health problems when compared to other adolescents (Mental Health Foundation 2002).

For example, 50% of young people detained in the Youth Treatment Service at Glenthorne Centre (a Department of Health facility that closed in 2000 which provided secure accommodation to some of Britain's most challenging young people) reported mental health problems that justified professional input (Bhatti *et al.* 1996). Another study that screened 192 young offenders (age range 10–17 years) attending a city-centre Juvenile Court in Manchester found that 15% had recent contact with psychiatric services, 10% had recent psychology contact, 11% had a head injury, 9% had a history of deliberate self-harm, 23% engaged in high-risk behaviours, 42% used alcohol, 10% used solvents and 38% used cannabis (Dolan *et al.* 1999). Similarly, a survey of 73 young offenders (age range 12–17 years) in contact with Warwickshire Youth Offending Services found that 55% had sustained a head injury, 86% used alcohol, 77% used illicit drugs, 26% had anger control problems, 49% reported a traumatic experience, 34% reported depression, 37% reported feelings of pessimism and hopelessness, 26% had anxiety-related problems and 8% had psychotic experiences (Warwickshire Youth Offending Service 2002). There is also convincing evidence that a significant proportion of young offenders have been victims of physical, sexual and emotional abuse (Boswell 1995).

Recently, the Policy Research Bureau (commissioned by the Mental Health Foundation) reported that, based upon their review of the existing literature, the prevalence of mental health problems for young people in contact with the criminal justice system ranges from 25% to 81%, with rates being highest for those in custody (Mental Health Foundation 2002). Their report also suggests that the rate of mental health problems in young offenders is three times as high as that for the general population.

Methodological difficulties, however, make it difficult to interpret some of the research findings. For example, whilst studies conducted in the United Kingdom and North America have focused upon similar aspects of mental health, they have employed different methods for assessing the presence and severity of problems. Some studies used clinical rating scales rather than specific psychometric instruments. Since most studies have involved participants who are in custodial settings and/or receiving treatment, the existing literature largely neglects those young offenders with potentially unmet needs. In addition, few studies have included non-offender control groups, making it difficult to determine to what extent problems are specific to young offenders.

Despite the methodological problems inherent in the existing research, it can be safely concluded that young offenders are an at-risk population for mental health difficulties, many coming from troubled family backgrounds characterised by poverty, unemployment, inconsistent and erratic parenting, over-harsh discipline, and alcohol and substance misuse in family members, all of which are risk factors for both mental health problems and anti-social behaviour. Furthermore, it is also recognised that the act of offending itself may cause mental health problems (e.g. witnessing trauma and violence). Interactions with the criminal justice system are also stressful, particularly those associated with custody.

## Meeting mental health needs within youth offending teams

One issue that has caused considerable debate and consternation in YOTs in recent times is the introduction of a two-stage mental health screening programme by the YJB. Stage one involves administering a brief screening questionnaire covering a range of commonly found difficulties, including depression, anxiety, psychotic features and substance misuse. It is designed for use by any YOT worker with minimal mental health training and scored in such a way that it should identify young people requiring stage two of the assessment process. This comprises a more in-depth assessment (a semi-structured interview) which should be completed by the YOT health worker.

This new programme was introduced in the spring of 2003 and has been subject to widespread criticism for a variety of reasons (e.g. absence of research investigating the psychometric properties of the stage one screening tool; likelihood of identifying too many false-positives). Of particular concern to YOT health workers, however, are the implications for their workload. Many workers do not relish the prospect of spending excessive amounts of time administering second-stage interviews, fearing that it will either prove unnecessary or that needs will be identified that cannot be met due to lack of time and resources.

There is also concern that local CAMHS will not be able to offer support. The policies and practices of some CAMHS are not conducive to working with young offenders. For example, some services do not accept referrals for young offenders, whilst others exclude young people with a history of violence. It is well recognised that provision for young people aged 16–18 years with mental health problems is inadequate as they fall between child and adult services. Given that offending rates peak around the age of 16 years, it is a crucial time to intervene. Increasing numbers of 16–17 year-olds on YOTs (and CAMHS) caseloads are being passed on to adult mental health services that are ill-equipped to adequately address the complex needs of 'reluctant-to-engage' adolescents. This may change in light of the expected proposals in the new National Service Framework for Children whereby CAMHS change their upper age limit to 18 years (Department of Health 2003).

Recent performance measures set by the YJB include six objectives focusing upon CAMHS providing rapid-response assessments for those young people identified by YOTs as manifesting mental health difficulties. However, this is rarely achieved, with long waits for CAMHS of up to a year tending to be the norm nationally and increasing numbers of young people being referred to adult forensic mental health services. Whilst this is unacceptable, it is often the only means for securing a speedy response from local mental health services. Clearly, these difficulties fly in the face of the YJB's expectation that close links should exist between YOTs and CAMHS.

## Consulting with youth offending teams

In light of the issues raised above, it is perhaps not surprising that some YOTs have sought consultation from external mental health agencies. In some instances the use of consultation services has been viewed by YOT managers as necessary to the development of the team, whilst in others it has been sought only in response to persistent lobbying from YOT practitioners. The authors' own experiences suggest that YOT practitioners are required to work with a significant number of extraordinarily complex and difficult young people. Furthermore, some of these youngsters present with a range of deeply entrenched behavioural and mental health difficulties set against a background of long-term family, educational and community/neighbourhood problems. Where the young person has also com-mitted serious offences, sometimes of a worrying and disturbing nature, it is little wonder that YOT workers feel they could do with all the help and support they can get.

To date, consultation arrangements with YOTs have been developed on an *ad hoc* basis.

Some YOTs have access to well-established mental health resources, whilst others operate in isolation, limited by the absence of local suitable resources. Both authors are currently involved in consulting with YOTs, using different models of working developed according to local need. One author consults with a group of health practitioners working in two different YOTs in a county-wide service. The consultancy arrangement is viewed as primarily fulfilling a need for continued professional development, at both an individual and team level. The team members expressed a strong desire to build and develop their knowledge and expertise as health workers within YOTs, whilst at the same time exploring the professional, statutory and political context in which YOTs operate. Meanwhile, the second author consults with all members of a YOT about cases they are involved with (as will be outlined in more detail later).

In both instances, the consultancy work began with a meeting with the YOT managers and practitioners, with the aim of clarifying the nature of the consultancy arrangement and agreeing terms and conditions of the working relationship. In developing a consultancy relationship it is important to consider a number of critical issues, discussed below.

## Nature of the relationship between the consultant and the YOT

The term 'consultancy' has a variety of different meanings. Consequently, members of the YOT may well have expectations that are different to that of the consultant. Failure to spend time discussing and clarifying the role of the consultant can have disastrous consequences. The model of consultancy advocated in the present chapter is one in which the consultant embarks on a process of helping the consultees, in this instance YOT workers, to achieve individual and team objectives. There are several critical features to this relationship, outlined below.

## Mutual collaboration

The process of consultation is construed as a collaborative exercise in which both parties are on a learning curve and both bring expertise, skills and knowledge to the task. The consultant's primary role is one of facilitation, informed by an understanding of the work carried out within YOTs, with the aim of helping the team to meet its objectives. Within this model the consultant is not an all-seeing, all-knowing 'expert' with the task of telling how others should do their jobs. The skill of the consultant lies in helping the team (or part of the team) to solve its own difficulties, such that team members develop new knowledge and skills along the way and retain responsibility for their decisions and actions.

This approach has been described by Caplan (1970, 1995) and Steinberg (1989) and sharply contrasts with the approaches reported across the existing published literature on mental health professionals providing consultation in forensic settings. Elsewhere, consultants are typically seen as 'experts' being called upon to advise the Courts (e.g. Jaffe *et al.* 1985; Lamb *et al.* 1996), police (e.g. Dodson-Chaneske 1989; Lamb and Weinberger 1998), staff in secure settings (e.g. Leschied *et al.* 1989) and others involved with criminal justice systems (e.g. Barnum 1993; Fritz *et al.* 1993; Coggins and Pynchon 1998) on issues relating to mental health and offending.

Mutual collaboration is always more straightforward when the consultant's role is solely restricted to the process of consultation. It becomes more complex when the consultant also undertakes direct clinical work with young offenders. In this *dual role* the consultant will be conscious of 'wearing two hats': one in which the primary role is to use the consultation process to help the YOT workers fulfill their own objectives (a facilitative function), the other in which they act in a clinical role, taking on case-work for which they assume some degree of professional and clinical responsibility. These two roles are very different (i.e. *consultancy by the consultant* is distinct from *clinical work by the consultant*) and can create conflict between the YOT and the consultant, as in the example presented below.

---

**Case study 9.1 Expectations about the consultant–consultee relationship**

In the consultancy role, the consultant and the YOT manager agreed that specific types of work fell within the remit of the YOT, notably assessment of reoffending risk. However, the YOT workers themselves felt that they lacked skills in this area and decided to refer young people to the consultant for a clinical 'assessment of risk'. With the agreement of the YOT manager, the consultant agreed to undertake training and skill development with a view to helping the YOT workers undertake this work themselves. The consultant duly provided this training through a process of mutual collaboration, with YOT workers taking on specific learning tasks, contributing to the training

---

*Continued*

process and providing case material for discussion, with oversight and guidance from the consultant.

   Nevertheless, following completion of the training programme, the YOT workers continued to lack confidence in their risk assessment work and insist that the consultant continued to accept case-work referrals. The consultant, however, was reluctant to get involved on the basis that risk assessment fell within the remit of the YOT, thereby creating a source of tension between the two parties. It was important to resolve these differ-ences as soon as possible by a process of negotiation, with the team members, manager and the consultant all involved in this process.

Generally speaking, these types of conflicts and tensions can be resolved. With reference to the above example, it may be possible to reach an agreement in which certain types of cases are suitable for referral to the consultant (e.g. offenders and offences with unusual characteristics), with some cases first being discussed in consultancy meetings to decide on the best course of action. However, in other instances, tension and conflict may continue, creating resentment and undermining the consultancy relationship. In these types of situation the quality of the consultant's relationship with the YOT manager and with YOT workers will have a significant influence on how, or whether, the conflict can be resolved. It may be necessary, for example, to convene a meeting with the YOT manager to discuss the difficulties, hopefully as early as possible to prevent the conflict escalating.

## Professional boundaries, responsibility and accountability

Whilst the consultant may well help the team to debate specific issues, it is vital that decisions are owned by the team and by individual practitioners and not by the consultant.

   Failure to adhere to professional boundaries can result in a range of difficulties, including confusion about lines of professional responsibility and accountability for case-work. This is illustrated in the example presented below.

### Case study 9.2  Confusing the lines of responsibility

Decisions in Court were delayed because the Judge was convinced that the YOT consultant was ultimately responsible for a case-work decision, even though the consultant was not directly involved in any clinical case-work with the YOT. The consultant was directed to attend the hearing and questioned about matters on which he was unable to comment. This kind of confusion can have damaging legal consequences for the consultant (e.g. in cases of alleged negligence or malpractice). It can also undermine the confidence and skills of the YOT practitioner, who may feel usurped and de-skilled by the consultant because other professionals seek the views of the consultant in preference to their own.

## Case-work supervision

The issue of case-work responsibility is particularly pertinent to case-work supervision. Consultants are often approached to undertake case-work supervision (e.g. to help YOT workers deal with particularly complex cases, or to develop skills in relation to specific types of problems such as fire-setting). However, the term 'supervision' has many different meanings, one of which implies line-management responsibility. Indeed, this is how the term is used in most hierarchical organisations, with each supervisor having professional responsibility for work carried out by junior staff, including setting performance targets, providing regular feedback and appraisal, and setting professional development targets. These types of supervisory arrangements are present in all YOTs, with each practitioner (at least in principle) having access to a line manager within their parent profession. It is therefore essential that consultants avoid being placed in a position where their work is confused with line-management supervision.

The consultant should be clear about lines of professional responsibility and should arrive at an agreement with the YOT manager and practitioners when setting up the consultancy contract. All parties should understand that some issues are to be dealt with only through line-management supervision, including those with statutory requirements (e.g. child protection concerns). The onus is on both the consultant and the YOT workers to understand and adhere to these professional rules of conduct. To avoid confusion, it is probably desirable to avoid the term 'supervision' within the consultancy arrangement. This does not mean that individual cases cannot be discussed, or that more formal 'clinical supervision' cannot be provided. It is simply necessary to be clear about the nature and description of this work and to ensure that line-management supervisors are kept informed of any significant developments. For example, the YOT group and the consultant may agree to have a regular slot within their meetings for case presentations and discussion ('case-work consultancy'), in which all members of the meeting can take an active part in the discussion, make comments and provide suggestions. Some members of the group may have expertise in relation to specific types of work and may well take a lead in the discussion. Occasionally, a YOT worker may wish to bring the same case for discussion to successive meetings, with the aim of tracking progress and developments and seeking ongoing support and guidance from the group. Another scenario is that the consultant agrees to provide teaching or training on a specific topic (e.g. sexual offending in adolescents), perhaps at the suggestion of the YOT worker or the YOT manager. As noted earlier, case-work responsibility and accountability remain with the YOT worker and their line manager, *except* in cases in which the consultant is directly clinically involved, such that the consultant assumes the usual level of clinical and professional responsibility for his or her work.

## Confidentiality

The content of discussions about individual young people and their families (YOT clients), some of which is of a highly sensitive nature (e.g. information about sexual abuse, unproven allegations of criminal behaviour, family relationships), should remain confidential within the boundaries of the group (i.e. the YOT workers and the consultant present at the meeting). Where a decision is made by a YOT worker to take a specific course of action in relation to a young person, the decision is owned by the worker and is passed on through the usual lines of communication within the YOT and other involved agencies within the usual YOT boundaries of confidentiality. Using the consultation group in this way provides a safe and secure forum for frank and honest discussion in which group members can learn from their practice and seek support and guidance without fear of looking foolish: one of the most important themes is the idea that there is no 'expert'. All participants are on a learning curve with varying degrees and depths of understanding about specific topics, such that the degree of 'expertness' is always relative depending on group composition and the issue being addressed.

The exception to this general rule is where information is disclosed to the consultant indicating that an individual is at risk of significant harm and where no member of the YOT group will agree to take action. Consider the scenario presented in the case study below.

---

**Case study 9.3  Boundaries of confidentiality**

The team believed that a professional colleague, who was not a member of the consultancy group, was placing himself at risk during visits to the home of a client known to have a history of serious and unprovoked violence. The worker had been advised against visiting the home but continued to do so, unbeknown to his line manager, on the basis that he was acting in the client's best interest. Members of the YOT consultancy group felt unable to alter their colleague's behaviour and were wary of reporting him to his manager because he was a senior, respected figure. Therefore, they approached the consultant to make their views known to the YOT manager.

---

## Content and themes of consultancy

YOT workers and managers may seek consultancy for a variety of reasons, some of which have been alluded to earlier. Skills and knowledge development, 'case-consultancy' to help with particularly complex or worrying cases, and team functioning within the context of political, legislative and policy changes are usually high on the agenda. Team members may seek help with specific issues, perhaps related to their own professional and personal development goals (e.g. to develop a risk-assessment policy for violent offenders). It is generally a useful strategy to begin the consultancy relationship with a broad set of aims and objectives in order to avoid being tied into a narrow framework and to allow YOT workers to develop their own agenda according to need and preference. As noted earlier, it is important to develop a collaborative relationship: in the consultancy role, the consultant's task is to facilitate learning, development and problem-solving and not to do the work of the team. Some team members may expect the consultant to provide 'ready-made' solutions and may be disappointed to find that they are required to do much of the work themselves!

## Frequency and location of consultancy sessions

Finally, agreement needs to be reached on the practical matters of where to meet and how often. With respect to location, this can prove to be a significant issue because some YOTs are county-wide, covering a wide geographical area. Some cities and regions have more than one team, each covering a specific geographical area, but with different parts of the team (e.g. health workers) using the same consultant. It may be necessary to rotate the venue for meetings or perhaps meet at the most central, convenient venue. It usually helps to have access to visual aids such as an overhead projector and flip-chart and to meet in a room that is relatively informal and conducive to group discussion. The frequency of meetings will depend on the needs of the team and the type of consultancy agreed in the consultancy contract. Where training and team development are the main priorities, monthly or even bi-monthly meetings will probably be sufficient. However, YOTs that require the consultant to provide regular case-work consultancy or to accept clinical case-work referrals via the YOT or to provide a referral route to local CAMHS (for instance, where the consultant is contracted in from local NHS services) will benefit from having more frequent contact with the consultant, probably on a weekly basis.

# Consultancy in practice: the South Staffordshire service

## The local picture: setting the scene

The consultant was approached by the local YOT to consider ways of meeting their needs. In the first instance, he attended two meetings with the YOT. The meetings were attended by all YOT practitioners who raised various concerns about the provision of mental health services to young offenders in the local area.

Historically, the YOT had been unable to secure a rapid response from their local CAMHS teams due to lengthy CAMHS waiting lists. Given the YOT health worker's generic role within the team, they had been finding it difficult to assess all young people referred with a mental health concern. Accordingly, their ability to devise and implement interventions for young people with mental health problems had become increasingly restricted.

Links between YOTs and CAMHS had been limited. It was evident during the meetings that the YOT practitioners were poorly informed about the work of CAMHS. Specifically, they were unsure about referral criteria, who to refer to, how to construct a referral, what information to include in the referral, and how referrals are prioritised and allocated within CAMHS. The YOT also raised concerns about the different style of working within CAMHS, particularly the clinic, appointment-based approach which they feared would result in most young people failing to attend and therefore not being engaged with services. The YOT practitioners, in common with other YOTs, had adopted an 'assertive outreach' approach, often visiting young people at home or at other more convenient venues, and were more flexible in arranging appointment times to suit the young person and their family/carers. The YOT also expressed a concern that they would receive little or no feedback from CAMHS about contact they had with young people referred by the team, partly based on a belief that CAMHS would consider their information to be confidential. In addition, the YOT believed that CAMHS tended to neglect the needs of young offenders and did not attach priority to YOT referrals. The consultant also discovered that the YOT had their own anxieties about how CAMHS viewed them. For example, they were concerned about being viewed as demanding and difficult, perceived by CAMHS as trying to jump waiting lists and unfairly requesting feedback.

Towards the end of the first meeting, the consultant asked the team what they would find most helpful. The practitioners overwhelmingly asserted that they were not trying to 'pass cases on'. Instead they were keen to work with the young people themselves and would value support in understanding more about mental health issues, how these impact upon a young person's life and how to best meet their needs. The YOT practitioners spoke clearly about their desire to enhance their own knowledge base as well as increase a young person's ability to engage with the YOT.

They envisaged receiving help on two levels. Firstly, to support all YOT workers with cases where mental health issues are evident. The team hoped this would assist the practitioners involved with planning and implementing interventions (aimed at reducing offending and enhancing social inclusion), thereby reducing the demands being placed upon the YOT health worker. Secondly, to provide support to the health worker in the team who is actively involved with many complex cases. Overall, the team wanted to make the most of the limited mental health resources available locally.

It was clear from the meetings that the YOT workers valued the role of the health worker and the work of CAMHS. Team members appeared to feel competent and confident enough to carry out some work with support and were able to recognise the need to refer some young people on for more specialist support. YOT workers also commented that some degree of stigma is, unfortunately, associated with referral to mental health services. Consequently, they would rather provide as much help as possible to young people within their own service to reduce the need to refer young people on to external mental health services.

## Setting boundaries: time and space

Following on from the initial meetings, the consultant agreed to set up a consultancy service with the YOT and to set aside time for what was termed 'mental health consultation clinics'. It was agreed that they would take place one morning fortnightly for a period of three hours. Meeting times were initially scheduled for a six-month period.

A procedure was set up whereby the health worker reminded the YOT workers of the next consultation clinic at the weekly team meeting and took note of who wanted to attend and the nature of any specific issues. It was agreed that the health worker would meet alone with the consultant for the first 60 minutes of each clinic to allow for case-work discussion. Typically, for the remainder of the morning, other team members would then join the consultant and the health worker to discuss cases they were involved with.

This system has proven to be very effective, with the health worker developing an oversight of the work of all YOT workers and gaining experience of the consultant's approach to various mental health issues. With respect to Caplan's (1970, 1995) model of consultation, the health worker provides the role of the 'stable person', with the ability to act as a channel for communication with other team members, become familiar with process issues, dispel concerns or prejudices raised from other team members, and promote appropriate use of the consultant and local mental health resources.

When practitioners request private discussions with the consultant, they confirm this with the health worker in advance. Typically, such meetings take place later in the morning. Given the nature of YOTs work (i.e. short-term interventions, high turnover of cases), new referrals arrive for allocation at each weekly team meeting. This emphasises the need for an open and flexible clinic setting.

The consultation clinics take place in a large meeting room (booked for the morning) in the YOT base. This ensures space, comfort and privacy. The room is large, which is important in light of the potential size of attendance. Whilst a typical consultation involves the consultant, health worker and another worker, on several occasions a group of practitioners involved with a case have attended (i.e. on one occasion four additional workers attended).

## Focus of consultation clinics

During the second meeting, the consultant and YOT formulated an agreement about the nature and style of the consultation process. Caplan (1970, 1995) defined four types of consultation:

| Type of consultation | Primary goal |
|---|---|
| client-centred | to help the client |
| consultee-centred | help the consultee to help the client |
| programme-centred administrative | to develop a treatment programme |
| consultee-centred administrative | help consultee develop a treatment programme |

It was agreed that the clinics comprise client-centred and programme-centred consultation, with the young people being the primary focus. Whilst many discussions have inevitably comprised a mixture of all four types of consultation, it is useful to remain aware of the primary aims and focus. This framework is discussed in consultation reviews that take place each six months. At the time of writing the consultation clinics have been running for almost one year and one review has taken place. Setting regular reviews ensures evolution and provides time for the practitioners and the consultant to reflect upon the clinics, share feedback, assess changes and consider strengths and difficulties.

## Evolution: adaptation and survival of the fittest

For the first six months of the service, YOT practitioners expressed concerns about how to best use the time allocated for the clinics, how to identify appropriate cases for discussion and how to set the agenda (i.e. what to talk about). The consultant referred to the notion of 'evolution', in the sense that the process will evolve itself, the most important and helpful things will remain, and that there are no right and wrongs. The consultant highlighted that the clinics are about providing time and space to think and reflect upon the work of the YOT and that the regular reviews will help shape the format of meetings in the longer term.

## The 'consulting with YOTs' philosophy

Another theme to address early on was sharing the underlying philosophy: the notion of consulting *with* YOTs as opposed to 'for' or 'to'. These are fine distinctions, but important nevertheless. The aim was to use the model of consultation advocated by Caplan (1970, 1995) and Steinberg (1989) in which the emphasis is on joint exploration of issues and mutual learning and development. The consultant did not want the YOT to be a passive recipient of his 'expertise'. Rather, he wanted to work collaboratively *with* the YOT, with both parties accepting that they can learn from each other. The consultant, whilst bringing to the clinics psychological and consultancy knowledge and skills, was keen not to be viewed as knowing everything about the work carried by YOTs. It would take time to build up a shared understanding of each other's perspective and to establish an effective working relationship in which the skills and expertise of both parties were used to maximum benefit.

From the perspective of the consultant, the initial impression was one of feeling 'what can I offer?' The YOT workers are dealing with complex cases within a complex multi-agency, multidisciplinary framework. Many of the workers are very experienced and skilled, working to a high professional standard within a statutory framework. The consultant took the view that he had to manage his own anxiety and apprehension and to be open and honest about the gaps in his knowledge and understanding, rather than pretend that he was an all-knowing, all-seeing expert.

Creating an 'illusion' of being an expert is not helpful for a number of reasons. For example, YOT workers would assume a level of knowledge and would not attempt to explain their work to the consultant. In turn, the consultant would feel unable to ask simple questions, not wanting to be seen as ignorant and inexperienced. The long-term consequence of beginning the consultancy relationship in this manner is that the learning curve builds on fragile foundations, with large gaps in understanding that can result in poor decision making. Declaring one's ignorance in the first meeting can be an enlightening experience, enabling one to ask any ridiculous-sounding question! Admitting to ignorance is much more difficult later in the consultancy relationship when YOT workers will be unimpressed and even dismayed by the consultant's lack of understanding, perhaps construing this as a lack of interest in their work.

## Confidentiality

It was agreed that all information remains private and confidential to those present at the meeting. However, the consultee continues to be responsible for sharing case-work concerns discussed within the consultation meeting with other agencies as and when required (e.g. child protection concerns).

The need to be clear about issues of confidentiality is important for a number of reasons. For example, YOT workers may be anxious about sharing information with the consultant because they fear that information will be passed on to their line managers. Discussion about this issue early in the consultancy process can be reassuring to YOT workers, helping to develop a more open and constructive working relationship.

The consultant also needs to be wary of confidentiality when keeping records of consultancy meetings. In South Staffordshire during case discussions, the consultant records the young person's details (i.e. name, date of birth, address and GP details) and details of the consultation (i.e. consultee details, duration of discussion, brief details of discussion) on a 'Record of Consultation' document. This document is placed in a consultation file held by CAMHS – accordingly, each young person discussed is allocated a case number with CAMHS.

## Consultant's availability

Decisions were made about availability of the consultant between meeting times. This is less of an issue where the role of the consultant is primarily one of training and development. However, owing to the consultant's role in providing case-work consultancy and support to the YOT, he agreed to be available outside of clinic times during weekday working hours. The consultant felt there was a need to be seen as approachable and contactable. Indeed, at the first review, practitioners stated that it was particularly useful to have a single point of contact when concerns arise about mental health issues. The consultant has been contacted outside clinic times on only a handful of occasions. On those occasions, a brief discussion took place and it was agreed that further discussion should take place at the next clinic. The consultant's input seems to serve as a safety net in addressing practitioners' concerns.

## Clinical and professional responsibility

It was agreed that professional responsibility remains with the consultee in that they accept or reject the help and advice given by the consultant. As noted earlier in the chapter, consultees should receive support, supervision and guidance from their professional manager/supervisor.

One assumption underpinning the consultation agreement is that the consultees are competent professionals who are able to recognise difficulties in their work and put into place action plans to remedy difficulties, such as a need for further training or supervision (e.g. see Steinberg 1989, p. 105). Both the YOT manager and health worker are aware of which team members attend the clinics. In the role of the 'stable' team person, the health worker can support and guide those involved with the clinics outside the consultations.

Case study 9.4 illustrates some of the ways in which the boundaries between the role of the consultant and the consultee may become blurred, raising issues about clinical and professional responsibility and the need to be clear about such matters.

---

**Case study 9.4 The boundaries of consultation**

Peter had been charged with a serious physical assault. Based on discussion with the YOT workers, there was reason to suspect that he presented with features of post-traumatic stress (e.g. nightmares, flashbacks, exaggerated startle response, hyperarousal). Upon inspection of his records, these difficulties appeared to stem from two incidents: one in which he witnessed

---

*Continued*

his brother being killed in a hit-and-run incident, the other in which he was the victim of a vicious assault. Subsequent to these incidents, Peter began to drink more and more, which the consultant suggested was an attempt to reduce the painful thoughts and memories resulting from the traumatic incidents. It was also hypothesised that he was at increased risk of becoming violent since he experienced intense feelings of anger (about the loss of his brother and being the victim of violence) and was in a state of heightened arousal when in public (relating to the post-traumatic stress). He committed the offence when intoxicated, raising the possibility that he was most at risk for reoffending when he had been drinking. During the consultation, the YOT practitioners were keen to secure a speedy response from CAMHS and local alcohol services and asked for the direct intervention of the consultant to liaise with CAMHS. In this instance the consultant agreed to this course of action, moving beyond his usual consultative role into a clinical role. Part of the consultation meeting was used to telephone the local CAMHS during clinic time and to construct a referral letter. By liaising with other professionals, the consultant became directly involved in the case and assumed a level of clinical case responsibility for this piece of work.

## Emerging themes from the consultation clinics

A number of themes emerged in the consultancy clinics held in the first few months.

### Continuity

For the consultant involved, the clinics may be unpredictable – which can generate a mixture of enthusiasm, excitement and intense anxiety for him each Wednesday morning! Until the clinic begins, he has no idea what issues will arise and who he will meet that day. Several weeks may pass between meetings with a practitioner who has brought a case for discussion. From this, the consultant may sometimes feel that practitioners are dipping in and out of the process and wonder whether practitioners are investing sufficient time and energy into the clinics or fully 'owning' the process. Whilst the consultant may have had some of these concerns when the clinics began, he did not fully appreciate how busy the team is – this was duly highlighted and discussed at the six-month review. Indeed, the very thing the YOT practitioners value from the clinics is having an 'open-door, as and when' policy.

   Given the lengthy time lapses between meetings with some of the consultees, it is difficult to pick up issues from where they were left previously. Furthermore, the consultant is often left wondering how cases are progressing in between times in the absence of further discussions. Since the consultant is not the practitioner's line manager or supervisor, it is inappropriate to track cases unless the practitioner brings them to the clinics. In South Staffordshire, the consultant usually makes brief enquiries about the progress of cases with practitioners he has consulted with previously – this assists with the ethos of mutual collaboration and demonstrates a genuine interest on the part of the consultant.

## Taking time out to think

Because the YOT is so busy with heavy case-loads, it is understandably difficult for practitioners to take time out to discuss specific issues. The modern pressures of accountability, securing the required number of contacts and meeting objectives and performance targets add to the pressure of being seen to be 'doing' things. The consultees have often stated that they rarely have the chance to stop and think about their work. In their opinion, the many directives and new initiatives set by the YJB over the past two years have prevented the team from reflecting upon their practice and consolidating gains and progress made. Furthermore, it is challenging and emotionally demanding and upsetting to think about the complex issues relating to young people who have usually experienced significant childhood trauma. One psychology colleague often talks about mental health services, organisations and teams adopting characteristics of their client group. In the case of youth offending, one may suggest that the client group comprises young people who have 'acted without thinking'. The authors wonder whether, at times, YOTs are in danger of doing this – something the consultant has recently brought into clinic meetings for consideration with consultees.

## The mystery of mental health

YOT workers vary in their knowledge and experience of mental health issues. Some workers felt apprehensive about dealing with mental health issues, commenting that 'I'm not trained in mental health', 'I'm out of my depth', 'what do we do with dual diagnoses?' and 'I'm only trained in drugs and alcohol'. One of the functions of the consultation clinics has been to demystify the concept of mental health, with an emphasis on constructing problems within a psychological framework; for example, separating the behaviours from the young person, discussing the notion of individual differences and viewing young people's difficulties in terms of their life experiences and as lying upon a continuum of presentations (as opposed to using restrictive diagnostic terms).

## The 'quick fix'

YOT workers came to the initial consultancy clinics armed with a list of questions and requests. Frequently, these questions took the form 'Have you got anything on anger . . . or sex offenders . . . or fire-setting . . .?' The idea that there was a simple, 'off the shelf' solution to a particular problem was common, usually based on the belief that 'someone, somewhere' must have an answer. In light of the complexity of many of the cases, this is rarely true. One of the most important functions of the YOT consultant is to encourage workers to reflect on their work and to develop solutions commensurate to the problem in hand. Also, to be realistic and accept that some problems are long-standing, complex and persistent and will not respond quickly to interventions. Furthermore, the approach adopted in the clinics (i.e. one of mutual collaboration) helped overcome the apparent desire of practitioners to 'get things right with the expert' – the consultant was left with the impression that consultees were overly anxious in earlier meetings about using the time 'correctly' and arriving at the 'right answer' with the 'expert'.

### Reassurance seeking

Some workers were also keen to be reassured that they were 'doing the right thing'. Youth crime is a major political issue and everyone seems to have an opinion on how to deal with young offenders. YOT workers feel under pressure to provide an effective service and this inevitably leads to anxiety and self-doubt about performance. The YOT consultant provides an important source of support and reassurance, helping to boost confidence and providing a sounding board for workers to assess the validity of their work.

## Developing local services

An interesting by-product arising from the consultancy service has been a growing desire in recent months from the YOT and the local NHS trust to improve local mental health care for young people who have offended or who are at risk for offending. Other YOTs in the locality have requested that similar consultation clinics be set up. Accordingly, YOT managers are currently bidding for additional funding to extend the service across the region. Funding was secured for a time-limited 'assessment and intervention' clinic, set up and run as a pilot. Referrals were accepted from the YOT (sometimes directly from the consultation clinic) and the consultant provided psychological assessments, formulations and interventions for young people. This time-limited pilot enabled YOT requests to be responded to quickly and effectively, whilst also providing an inter-agency initiative to try to secure long-term funding for the clinic. A research grant was also awarded to investigate the prevalence of mental health problems among young offenders across the county.

These exciting initiatives stem from local CAMHS and YOT practitioners forging links, sharing their experiences and concerns, co-working and highlighting the unmet needs of young people who offend or who are at risk of offending. In some respects, the consultation clinic has been a catalyst for change locally.

## Conclusions and future directions

YOTs are a relatively recent innovation, bringing together a diverse range of professionals and disciplines to prevent offending among young people. It is becoming increasingly apparent that a significant proportion of young offenders have mental health problems and that traditional services have been unable to meet the needs of this population, many of whom have been excluded in one way or another from mainstream services. The inclusion of health workers within YOTs has drawn attention to this unmet need and the process of developing resources and professional networks to develop an effective mental health service is in its infancy. Professionals providing consultancy services to YOTs are in a privileged position of witnessing the transformation of youth offending services at first hand and have an opportunity to make a valuable contribution to this field of work. Mental health professionals who are new to working with young offenders are often surprised at the extent and severity of psychosocial problems in this population and the need to be creative in developing new services that are responsive to the needs of troubled adolescents. Future challenges include the need to develop service provision for older adolescent offenders in the 16–18 year range, many of whom fall between the gap that exists between child and adult services. The model of consultancy promoted by Caplan (1970, 1995) and Steinberg (1989) has utility in that it emphasises the need for YOTs to be responsible for their own growth and development, using external consultancy services as and when necessary to help solve problems, build and develop skills and foster links with other services. Many YOTs are now in a position to begin commissioning research, looking not only at service-related issues (e.g. referral pathways, outcomes and intervention effectiveness) but also theoretical questions that have hitherto been neglected (e.g. the relationship between head injury and offending in young people, the prevalence of mild learning difficulties and autism spectrum features in young offenders). It is likely that mental health professionals providing consultancy to YOTs will play a significant role in helping to develop this research and development agenda.

# References

Audit Commission. *Misspent Youth*. Audit Commission, London, www.auditcommission. gov.uk.

Barnum R (1993) An agenda for quality improvement in forensic mental health consultation. *Bulletin of the American Academy of Psychiatry and the Law*. **21** (1): 5–21.

Bhatti V, Vostanis P, Lengua C et al. (1996) *Establishment of Need for the Development of Child and Adolescent Forensic Services in Birmingham*. South Birmingham Mental Health Trust, Birmingham.

Boswell G (1995) *Violent victims: the prevalence of abuse and loss in the lives of Section 53 offenders*. The Prince's Trust, London.

Caplan G (1970) *The Theory and Practice of Mental Health Consultation*. Tavistock Publications, London.

Caplan G (1995) Types of mental health consultation. *Journal of Educational and Psychological Consultation*. **6** (1): 7–21.

Coggins M and Pynchon MR (1998) Mental health consultation to law enforcement: Secret Service development of a mental health liaison program. *Behavioral Sciences and the Law*. **16** (4): 407–22.

Department of Health (2003) *Getting the Right Start: National Service Framework for Children – emerging findings*. Retrieved 1 August 2003 from www.doh.gov.uk/nsf/ children/emergingfindings.pdf

Dodson-Chaneske D (1989) Mental health consultation to a police department. *Journal of Human Behavior and Learning*. **5** (1): 35–8.

Dolan M, Holloway J, Bailey S et al. (1999) Health status of juvenile offenders: a survey of young offenders appearing before the juvenile courts. *Journal of Adolescence*. **22**: 137–44.

Fritz GK, Mattison RE, Nurcombe B et al. (1993) *Child and Adolescent Mental Health Consultation in Hospitals, Schools and Courts*. American Psychiatric Press, Inc., Washington, DC.

Jaffe PG, Leschied AW, Sas L et al. (1985) A model for the provision of clinical assessments and service brokerage for young offenders: the London Family Court Clinic. *Canadian Psychology*. **26** (1): 54–61.

Lamb HR, Weinberger LE and Reston-Parham C (1996) Court intervention to address the mental health needs of mentally ill offenders. *Psychiatric Services*. **47** (3): 275–81.

Lamb HR and Weinberger LE (1998) Deinstitutionalization: promise and problems. New directions for mental health services. *Psychiatric Services.* **49** (4): 483–92.

Leschied AW, Austin GW and Riley E (1989) Description and assessment of a crisis consultation program in a youth detention center. *Canadian Journal of Criminology.* **31** (2): 145–54.

Mental Health Foundation (2002) *The Mental Health of Young Offenders. Bright futures: working with vulnerable young people.* Mental Health Foundation, London.

Rutter M, Giller H and Hagell A (1998) *Antisocial Behaviour by Young People.* Cambridge University Press, New York.

Rutter M and Smith DJ (eds) (1995) *Psychosocial Disorders in Young People.* John Wiley and Sons, Chichester.

Steinberg D (1989) *Interprofessional Consultation.* Blackwell Scientific Publications, Oxford.

Warwickshire Youth Offending Service (2002) *Health Needs Analysis 2000–2001.* Prepared for North Warwickshire and South Warwickshire NHS Trusts.

Youth Justice Board (2002) *Youth Justice Board Review 2001/2002: building on success.* Youth Justice Board, London.

# Chapter 10

# Mental health provision through consultation to a local authority secure children's home

*Johanna Hilton*

## Introduction

This chapter focuses on the use of consultation as a framework for offering mental health provision to a local authority secure children's home. Secure children's home accommodation occupies a distinctive position among resources for children and young people. Whilst firmly located within residential child-care provision, it operates at the interface with the criminal justice system.

The chapter is divided into four sections. The first section of the chapter provides background information on secure homes, the criteria for placement and the types of young people who are accommodated in these settings.

The second section focuses on the particular mental health issues that this population is faced with and types of mental health provision offered within this context. In section three of the chapter, reference is made to a specific secure home, describing the development of the mental health provision chronologically. In particular it highlights, with case illustrations, the initial process of engagement leading to the establishment of a case-led consultation forum, in parallel with service development/organisational consultation. Some of the issues specific to working within a secure setting will be discussed, with a particular emphasis on considering the role and remit, within a mental health context, of the staff working on a daily basis with the young people.

In the fourth section the chapter then moves on to explore factors relating to offering a consultation provision in such a setting. The final part of the chapter highlights useful issues to consider when embarking on this type of work.

## Secure accommodation criteria, placement decisions and characteristics of the population

### Local authority secure children's homes

Also known as child secure units or local authority secure units, these establishments are governed by the Children (Secure Accommodation) Regulations made under Section 25 of the Children Act 1989. As at 31 March 2003, the National Statistics (Department for Education and Skills [DfES] 2003) indicate that there were 445 approved places in 31 secure units in England and Wales (*see* Table 10.1).

As the number of units implies, children are often placed out of county, often long distances away from their families and local services.

## Criteria for placement

### Welfare

Secure accommodation is provided for young people for reasons of welfare, generally between the ages of 10–18 years, in cases where the young person is deemed likely to cause serious injury to themselves or others if placed in other forms of accommodation. Young people can be placed directly from their family homes or from a looked-after placement such as a foster home or residential home. Secure accommodation is also provided for young people detained or remanded to local authority accommodation who have a history of absconding and are likely to abscond from any other type of accommodation; and if they do so, are likely to cause harm to others or suffer significant harm themselves.

### Offenders

Young people sentenced to serious offences may also be accommodated in secure accommodation. The Youth Justice Board (YJB) is responsible for purchasing and placing young people in such instances and setting the standards for these facilities. A custodial sentence is given when no alternative is appropriate due to the seriousness of the offence, the history of the offender, or the risk to the public. Secure accommodation is one of three forms of custody available to the YJB. The other two sections of the 'juvenile secure estate' are secure training centres and young offender institutions.

Young people are placed in any of the three custodial facilities when they are:

- *sectioned under Section 90/91 of the Powers of Criminal Courts (Sentencing) Act 2000 (which replaces Section 53 of the Children and Young Person Act 1933).* This is when a young person has committed a 'grave offence' such as murder or rape or those offences for which an adult would receive a sentence of 14 years or more. Such sentences can only be given by a Crown Court and the entire sentence is completed in custody. The release date for a young person sentenced under Section 90 is decided by the Home Secretary. The release date for a Section 91 sentence is set automatically.
- *under a Detention and Training Order (Crime and Disorder Act 1998).* These Orders sentence a young person to custody. The Order can be given to 12–17 year-olds. The length of sentence can be between four months and two years. The first half of the sentence is spent in custody whilst the second half is spent in

**Table 10.1** National Statistics as at 31 March 2003 – approved secure unit places in England and Wales

| No. of units | No. of places in England | No. of places in Wales | Total no. of places |
|---|---|---|---|
| 31 | 425 | 20 | 445 |

the community under the supervision of the youth offending team (YOT). A Detention and Training Order is only given by the Courts to young people who represent a high level of risk, have a significant offending history or are persistent offenders, and where no other sentence will manage their risk effectively. The seriousness of the offence is always taken into account when a young person is sentenced to a Detention and Training Order.

* *juvenile on secure remand (Section 23 (4) Children and Young Person Act 1969)*. Ten to eleven year-olds cannot be held in secure accommodation for longer than 28 days when remanded without a further remand hearing. The Order is enabling rather than prescriptive, and gives the local authority the power to place the young person in secure accommodation but does not require them to do so.

## Placement decisions for offenders

The decision where to place a young person who has offended is made on a case-by-case basis by the Youth Justice Board Placement Team (Youth Justice Board 2001*b*) in consultation with the YOTs. The use of the ASSET assessment (*see* Chapter 9) and any sentence reports are key to this process. These are updated during the young person's sentence and also form the basis for the discharge plan at the end of the placement.

The main factors that influence placement decisions are outlined by the Youth Justice Board (2001*b*) (*see* Box 10.1).

---

**Box 10.1 Factors influencing placement decisions**

* Vulnerability
* Need to make local placements
* Matching regimes to needs
* Needs arising from gender
* Other, such as separating co-offenders

---

Overall, secure accommodation focuses on young offenders aged between 12–14 years, girls up to the age of 16 years and 15–16 year-old boys who are assessed as vulnerable or those young people judged to be too vulnerable to be detained in prison service accommodation. Vulnerability encompasses factors such as physical and emotional maturity and propensity towards self-harm.

Prior approval for placing a child aged 13 or below in secure accommodation must be sought from the Secretary of State for Health. The local authority should first discuss the case with the Social Services Inspectorate.

From the latest National Statistics (DfES 2003) as at 31 March 2003, of those accommodated in secure units about three-quarters of the total were being accommodated by reason of their offending or alleged offending behaviour. The remaining children and young people had been admitted on a welfare basis (*see* Table 10.2).

**Table 10.2** National Statistics: reasons for accommodation within a secure unit

| 31 March 2003 | Section 23 (4) Remand | Section 90–92 Grave Crimes | Detention and Training Orders | Welfare | Total |
|---|---|---|---|---|---|
| No. of children | 55 | 80 | 175 | 110 | 420 |

## Characteristics of the young people in secure accommodation

As can be seen from Table 10.3, at 31 March 2003 a snapshot from the National Statistics (DfES 2003) reveals that a total of 420 children were accommodated in these units, compared with 340 at 31 March 1999, indicating that occupancy rates have been increasing since 1999.

**Table 10.3** National Statistics on occupancy rate within secure units for 31 March 1999 and 31 March 2003

| | 31 March 1999 | 31 March 2003 |
|---|---|---|
| Occupancy rate | 340 | 420 |

The number of children staying longer in secure units has also increased. A total of 120 of those 420 children have been accommodated for six months or more, indicating a 44% increase from the period in 1999 when the number was 80 (*see* Table 10.4).

At 31 March 2003, of the total number of children accommodated in secure units in England and Wales, 68% were boys and 32% were girls. With regard to age, there has been a slight downward shift in the ages of children in secure units between 1999 and 2003 such that 49% of all children in 2003 were aged 14 years or under, whereas in 1999 the equivalent figure was 46% (*see* Table 10.5).

**Table 10.4** National Statistics on length of stay in secure units for 31 March 1999 and 31 March 2003

| | 31 March 1999 | 31 March 2003 |
|---|---|---|
| Six-month stay or longer | 80 | 120 |

**Table 10.5** National Statistics on percentage of young people accommodated in secure units

| | Percentage of boys | Percentage of girls | Percentage under 14 years |
|---|---|---|---|
| 31 March 1999 | 71 | 30 | 46 |
| 31 March 2003 | 68 | 32 | 49 |

No statistics were available on ethnic origin. This is surprising as there is ongoing concern for the overrepresentation of black young people within the Youth Justice System. Recent data from NACRO (2004) indicate that according to the YJB data, 5.7% of the youth offending population are classified as black or black British but account for almost 15% of those remanded to custody or secure accommodation.

## Risk factors

It is now generally recognised that the cluster of risk factors that feature in the lives of children who pass through the child protection system, and who come into contact with the Youth Justice System, bear a high level of similarity (Youth Justice Board 2001c).

There is a high degree of overlap between the two populations found within a secure unit, as shown in Box 10.2.

---

**Box 10.2 Risk factors for secure accommodation**

- Living with families affected by drugs, alcohol or domestic violence
- Special needs or a disability (emotional and behaviour problems are the commonest cause of disability in children)
- Coming from highly mobile families
- Young people may also have experienced poor access to services owing to language or cultural barriers

---

Other features common both to child protection and secure unit populations include: socio-economic adversity, multiple family problems and breakdown, experience of trauma and abuse. Also there are marked increases in risk of accommodation with physical illness, developmental delay and low educational achievement.

## Summary

To summarise, the local authority secure children's homes house both males and females, aged between 10–18 years, on either welfare or justice grounds for periods between a matter of days through several years. As a result, children may be at one of a wide range of developmental stages and abilities. There are also likely to be gender and cultural issues. Although there is a considerable overlap between the populations in terms of risk factors, the two routes for placement hold widely varying philosophies and are managed by different agencies following their own policies and procedures. As a result, mental health practitioners working with this population need to be familiar with clinical issues and systems relating to both the forensic and looked-after children services.

# Mental health needs, and review of mental health provision to secure accommodation

## Mental health needs

In the general population mental health problems in children and young people have been found to occur in up to 25% of the population. In contrast, mental health difficulties experienced by looked-after children have been estimated at 67% (Department of Health 2000). Similarly, Hagell (2002) on behalf of the Policy Research Bureau commissioned by the Mental Health Foundation estimated the prevalence of mental health problems for children and young people within the justice system as ranging from 25% to 81%, the rate being highest for those in custody. Boswell (1998) found 91% of offenders had experienced both abuse and significant loss. Boswell likened the serious juvenile offender to a victim of post-traumatic stress disorder whose ability to control their behaviour is much reduced. The report also suggests that the rate of mental health problems in young offenders is three times as high as that for the general population.

Those problems are likely to persist in later life and are not often met by children's mental health services (Richardson and Joughin 2000). For this reason there has been a number of recent government policy documents to promote the mental well-being of children and young people, in particular targeting vulnerable populations such as those who are looked after and those involved in the youth justice system. The policies also promote the enhancement of partnership between agencies to provide an integrated common framework for assessment, intervention planning and review for all children in need (*see* Chapter 5).

## Mental health provision

The local authority secure children's homes focus on attending to the physical, emotional and behavioural needs of young people sent to them. They are intended to provide the young person with support tailored to their individual needs, and with this in mind have a high ratio of staff to young person and are generally small facilities ranging from five to 38 beds (Youth Justice Board 2001*a*).

Since 2000 it has been a YJB requirement that young people placed by them undertake seven hours a week 'offending behaviour' work, a relatively new field within secure units (Hobbs and Hook Consulting 2001). Having less experience of formal programmes, young people's secure units have been found to have a tendency to take a whole-system or positive parenting approach where positive behavioural change is promoted on a day-to-day basis. This is described as providing a more holistic, pro-social modelling approach that has some overlap with the welfare model.

Hobbs and Hook Consulting (2001) summarised the literature regarding aspects of effective intervention for offending behaviour as:

- targeting: the right offender should be on the right programme, which matches the level of risk they present and deals with the particular problems relating to their criminal behaviour
- cognitive/behaviour component: offending links with faulty thinking patterns, poor problem solving and decision-making abilities. Hobbs and Hook Consult-

ing highlighted the need to address links between beliefs and thoughts and behaviour
* skill based/social inclusion
* clarity of purpose, focusing on primary offending-related issues
* well-trained and enthusiastic workers
* monitoring and evaluation
* consistency
* length and intensity to make impact on behaviour.

Hobbs and Hook Consulting (2001) found that overall there was a lack of age-appropriate programmes that took account of the wide variance in developmental stages of the population, in particular the pre-adolescent age group. Rather, most were adapted from adult populations with little evaluation and costing of work. They also noted little attention to needs of girls or special education needs. The review also highlighted the very limited work with families, noting that units predominantly focused on encouraging and facilitating family visits only.

Hobbs and Hook Consulting recommended a shift in focus to direct intervention work with the young person and family. They noted a need for staff to have appropriate levels of skills and supervision and support of the mental health practitioner to ensure consistency. Training and the ethos of the institution were also highlighted as key components for effective interventions.

At the time of this work in 1999–2000 most intervention by mental health services was through psychiatric and occasionally psychological input to undertake assessments. These assessments did not appear to have been incorporated into care planning or fully shared with the staff, other than to be placed in the young person's file. The focus of the assessments was predominantly on risk rather than providing a formulation that highlighted need and direction for intervention. Any intervention work was undertaken from the unit staff's own initiative with little direction or support from other agencies (including the mental health services), little management and with no supervision.

Additional difficulties were quickly highlighted with planned intervention, including the uncertainty of the length of stay for the welfare children. For those on welfare there may be insufficient time for long-standing problems to be addressed, alongside the young person being potentially preoccupied with leaving and so having little motivation to engage. Similarly, links with the community were poor and often difficult to facilitate when the young person's place of origin was out of region; although for the youth justice population this was improving with the youth offending practitioner links. However, discharge decisions were made on the basis of the young person's performance within the secure environment, not the community. There were very limited reintroductions back into their community with the potential for readmittance being increased and along with it the sense of failure.

## Local case illustration engagement, case-led consultation and service development/organisational consultation to a secure children's home

### Consultation in context

#### The unit

The unit was located in a village away from any central facilities. It consisted of two independent living areas, each comprising a lounge, dining room and six bedrooms with *en suite* facilities; a bedroom for emergency admissions which was also used as a medical room; a secure garage through which children arrived; an internal courtyard; a gymnasium; and an education area comprising of three classrooms, an office and a large store cupboard. There was also a large meeting room which doubled as the visitors' room and therapy room. This and the unit manager's office were located away from the living areas, next to the front entrance.

The unit was able to accommodate 12 children in two living groups of six. At the time of the author's involvement the unit had only recently been opened and accommodated between three and eight children at any one time.

The purpose of the unit was to provide a secure, safe and homely environment. It aimed to provide high-quality, professional, safe care for children who are vulnerable and/or at risk to themselves or others, in order to enable them to develop inner controls, respect for themselves and others, and take responsibility for their actions. The unit came under the jurisdiction of the County Council Social Services Department with overall management by the Assistant Director, Children and Families who was based off site and a unit manager on site. There were high staffing levels with two deputy managers and 24 staff allocated to three teams, each led by a qualified social worker.

Staff were residential social workers and generally had wide-ranging levels of experience and qualification, although all staff were in the process of being trained to a minimum of NVQ Level 3. There was also a small teaching staff of five as well as a range of support services, including administrative staff and domestic staff.

#### Unit links

The unit had specific links with other services, including a general practitioner, paediatrics, child social workers, police, youth offending teams and the child's family of origin. The unit had also developed links with the local community child and adolescent mental health services (CAMHS), developing contracts for mental health input. However, these contracts remained more or less 'virtual': although agreed on paper, when the consultant took up the post no mental health provision was in evidence and all efforts to provide a service seemed to have been declined by the unit.

---

**Case study 10.1 Initial contact**

Prior to commencing contact with the unit, attempts to engage with it had been limited. CAMHS had not been called upon to provide any services and had felt that their initial offers of involvement had been rebuked.

The first contact was a meeting between the consultant and the unit manager, initiated by the consultant, part of whose remit was to provide a service to the unit. On arrival there was no record of the visit. However, it was agreed that the meeting would go ahead. A security check was undertaken, in keeping with the unit's security protocol, which required the consultant's coat, briefcase and any loose items to be placed in a locked holding facility. A personal alarm was provided, along with an escort to the manager's office, a few feet away from the entrance (which was separate to the main living area where the children were housed).

During this initial meeting it became apparent that there was uncertainty regarding the contractual agreement between the services, that problems with the fabric of the facility dominated the manager's thinking and that the manager was unclear as to whether any specialist mental health provision was warranted.

The experience was far from welcoming.

---

The consultant persisted with arranging several meetings with the unit manager, during the course of which it became clear that the manager had limited experience and understanding of this child population. It was this, rather than anything else, that had resulted in the manager's ambivalence. One ingredient of her ambivalence was anxiety. For example, despite asserting that the children in the unit had no mental health problems and just needed 'nurturing', she evidenced considerable anxiety through her use of language, oscillating between throw-away comments about arriving at work to 'find all my staff killed' and repeated assertions that the unit had no need of outside help for the children as 'all their needs would be met by a settled environment'. Exploration revealed previous negative experience with mental health services that the manager was keen to avoid.

Fortunately, the mental health provision was not left to chance or personal whim. The social services department was requesting that services be implemented as soon as possible. It was therefore agreed that the initial work undertaken would be to consult the unit manager and social services department jointly to clarify the contractual arrangements and role and remit of provision.

A number of points can be highlighted as a result of this initial phase of consultation with the unit manager:

- There is a diverse population accommodated in secure settings, including children accommodated on welfare grounds and young offenders, and staff can often feel anxious about how to address the needs of both populations simultaneously.
- It is important to clarify who are the clients and stakeholders (all interested parties).
- It is important to understand the motivating forces, beliefs and relationships

pertinent to the stakeholders, particularly those that have developed out of previous experiences of mental health services.
- Within these settings there is the potential for an ambivalent response by staff to the security aspect of the service, in terms of the overzealous administration of protocols and procedures as well as their disregard.
- It helps to find common language, accept and take into account the benefits and difficulties of previous mental health experiences, and to try to arrive at a new understanding of what you are able to offer; often practical examples can be helpful.

Without taking these factors into account, any attempts at offering consultation will be limited or even thwarted as all parties will either not agree or have a differing understanding of the provision.

## Second phase of contact

During the process of clarification there was a change in unit manager such that a temporary manager came into post for a six-month period. An agreement was therefore made with the new unit manager in conjunction with the social services department to continue the clarification process regarding the contractual arrangements and mental health provision. The consultant set about meeting all of the staff to obtain their views about the sort of provision they would see as helpful to them and to the young people in the unit. It was also agreed that, in order to gain a better understanding and familiarity with the unit, the consultant would attend the unit for a full day, shadowing members of staff and meeting the young people.

This phase highlights the importance of working with organisational change. All public sector services are in a constant state of change that necessitates repetition of liaison and reclarification and is therefore best viewed as a dynamic ongoing process.

## Initial staff consultation

Staff were initially met at a full staff meeting where it became apparent that they had been informed by their previous manager that the service had refused any provision! As a result, staff were initially very hostile and understandably angry. However, they were able, once given the space to express their anxieties and concerns, to focus on possibilities for current provision.

In particular the staff requested:

- crisis telephone contact
- consultation to discuss children with a mental health practitioner at a regular set time
- provision of assessment tools
- behaviour management
- support in developing a systematic care plan
- they also requested training but were unable to say in what areas.

---

**Case study 10.2 Familiarisation process**

On the day of the shadowing, the unit staff had forgotten the consultant was attending and had not timetabled the visit in the diary. The consultant observed that attendance at hand-over was variable, and information shared varied in level of detail with no clear protocol to be followed. There were no regular staff meetings and no specific direct time for key workers to spend with children in order to complete the initial assessment. There was neither group nor individual work. It also transpired that there were no written policies for the staff to follow and that they had not received supervision or training beyond mandatory training requirements.

---

Conversations with staff members provided valuable additional information about conditions, routines, perceptions of competency and general morale.

---

**Case study 10.2 contd.**

Staff also informed the consultant that previous experience and qualifications varied enormously among the staff members. There was also a high turnover of staff and a high level of agency workers at that time. Staff presented as dispirited although strongly committed to their allocated shift team.

The staff worked within a highly technological and secure environment, which involved them carrying mobile radios with which to speak with each other. The children remained in their rooms for long periods of time and were often spoken to through an intercom system.

---

There was very poor organisation within the unit and limited communications between staff and teams and few fora to share information. It was hardly surprising that the staff presented as dispirited and worked hard to develop informal support and a sense of belonging through their teams. However, this would appear to have further exacerbated the limited communications and consistency of approach across teams due to a competitive atmosphere. This left a lot of scope for the young people to split the staff.

---

**Case study 10.2 contd.**

The consultant noticed as part of the shadowing exercise that in their interactions with the young people the staff presented as having limited confidence in their decision making and appeared uncertain as to whether to share information. They also presented as inconsistent, for example the consultant was asked not to let the children know that she was a psychologist when she met them, as staff were very concerned that this would lead the children to think that they were 'mental'. However, whilst with the children the same staff then proceeded to ask lots of questions

---

*Continued*

> about psychology. Similarly, the staff presented as very aware of safety issues in terms of the daily routine, but this did not appear to translate into their interactions with the children. For example, they appeared at ease discussing information in front of the children, whether about other children or about their own personal circumstances.

The staff's presentation, although concerning, was understandable in terms of the limited management support they had experienced and the current state of leadership transition. Furthermore, their behaviour could be seen as a reflection of the very same issues and difficulties that the young people would be facing.

The lack of confidence in decision making and information sharing can be understood in terms of anxiety by the staff to provide a positive environment for the children and attempt to work with them without appropriate support, training and advice. These concerns grew out of a culture of blame where concern as to whether they had 'done the right thing' was uppermost.

## Case-led consultation fora

Following the review and familiarisation with the unit it was agreed with the unit manager and staff that a regular consultation forum would be available for staff to meet with the consultant to discuss any issues relating to their work with individual young people. From this it was envisaged that any training needs and service development issues would be highlighted and taken forward.

Implementation of the consultation forum was undertaken, following very similar methods as outlined by Sinclair and Epps in Chapter 9. Specifically, the consultation forum had the aim of providing a space for staff to come individually or as a group to discuss the direct work they were undertaking with the children in their key worker role. It was hoped that this would facilitate the development of the key worker role.

Following very poor attendance, it was agreed with the unit manager and staff that all key workers would use the forum to bring completed initial assessments to discuss the care plan for each young person and start to think about direct work to be undertaken with the child.

At the six-month review it became clear that the consultation provision continued to be poorly used. There appeared to be a number of factors that impacted on this:

- staff found it difficult to free themselves from other unit activities
- circulation of the dates did not appear to have occurred and dates appeared not to be recorded or checked by staff in the diary. As a result, staff had not prepared for or allocated time to utilise the consultation forum
- staff expressed anxiety at using the forum. They felt unclear of their key worker role and what constituted direct work and were concerned that the forum would highlight their errors which would be fed back to the unit manager
- staff who did attend consultation described feeling uncertain as to how to make use of the time and would attend without any particular focus.

The consultant suggested at this point that the consultation forum was not the most useful means of providing help. The consultation forum had highlighted, among other things, that the staff were not ready to make use of it. Rather, training in mental health and associated topics might be more appropriate, commencing with a focus on professional skills and the key worker role. It was agreed that the initial focus should be on communicating effectively with children and an introduction to behaviour management. The consultant recommended that this would be complemented by some limited direct clinical work with the young people: this could provide a more useful way of consulting with staff through case liaison and joint working. In this way, over time, it was expected that staff's understanding and experience of assessment, case management, care plans and psychological interventions would increase and that at this point it might be worth considering restarting the consultation fora.

With regard to direct work it was agreed that the consultant would offer psychological assessments of the young people and, where possible, this would be done jointly with the key worker. Together, they would develop a formulation of the client's presenting difficulties, which would be used to form the basis of their care plan, identifying areas to be addressed, by whom, with time frames for reviewing. These clinical reviews were seen as distinct to the statutory reviews.

---

**Case study 10.3 Simon, 11 years**

Simon, aged 11, had a long history of psychiatric involvement prior to coming to the unit. On initial assessment he presented as a very defended young man. Due to the large number of assessments that he had under-taken over the years, Simon had developed a script of his life, which, although including very distressing details of his experiences, enabled him to disengage from and be devoid of emotion.

However, Simon found the exploratory nature of the assessment difficult. In particular, when the consultant reflected on how he might have felt or experienced certain events, Simon became very agitated and angry, stating that he did not wish to discuss his experiences and demanding to leave the session early. Following this session, Simon stated that he did not wish to meet with the consultant again. As a result it was agreed that work would be undertaken indirectly with Simon through his key worker.

Each week the consultant met Simon's key worker and used the information from the initial assessment to develop a formulation from which the key worker could be facilitated in her direct work with him. Simon was aware of the meeting, which he was able to join. He chose not to participate in these meetings but always checked that the consultant had attended.

---

The consultant and the key worker drew on attachment theory in understanding Simon's self-reliant, distrusting and limited capacity to regulate his emotions. This appeared to be exacerbated by pathological distress resulting from trauma experiences in his earlier years. They therefore prioritised focusing on Simon's key worker developing a positive relationship with Simon through specific dedicated time for fun and enjoyment, which was led by Simon. This gave his key worker the opportunity to attend, praise, compliment and start to build trust within their relationship. Owing to the shift patterns in the unit, this proved difficult to achieve. However, with less frequent meetings between the key worker and Simon than originally planned, and the commitment and creative problem solving of the key worker, she managed to ensure that she was able to offer a regular, reliable and predictable time with Simon.

The key worker and consultant met weekly to review progress with Simon and over a period of weeks the key worker was able to report Simon becoming more relaxed, spontaneous and sustaining the activity for longer. The key worker also noted that Simon started to speak more freely about how he felt and what he thought about things not only in the here and now but also in relation to his previous experiences.

## Service development consultation

It was recognised that the unit culture, structure and functioning had an additional impact on the use of the consultation forum by staff. Furthermore, by this time a new permanent manager had taken up post and was, as yet, unfamiliar to the staff. It was agreed with the manager to undertake regular consultations directly with him regarding service development.

In determining how to utilise the consultation forum for service development, initial meetings were spent with the unit manager discussing a range of presenting difficulties, hopes and aims, alongside statutory requirements. The consultant facilitated these discussions, using reframing, summarising and reflecting. From these discussions a list of areas to address through consultation were identified and prioritised jointly. These were:

1 developing an ethos for the service within a therapeutic milieu. In particular, facilitating the manager to develop clarity in his vision for the service
2 development of a clear management structure alongside role specification and responsibilities for all staff
3 support with staff selection and recruitment
4 facilitating the management of stress and anxiety within staff through review of their working conditions, including shift patterns and the identification, development and maintenance of support structures including: meetings, debriefing, supervision and continued professional development
5 developing systematic care planning. In particular, use of the initial assessment to define needs and objectives for the individual child during their time at the unit, as well as discharge planning
6 facilitating the development of assessment, monitoring and evaluation systems for the children
7 developing links with external services and the community.

Although it was recognised that these were interrelated, it was agreed that each would be focused on in turn. Through consultation, the manager was offered the opportunity to clarify the current situation and explore alternative options. Mental health advice and research evidence was also available to help inform his thinking. It was also possible to explore different approaches for the manager to consult with his staff and the young people to obtain their views.

---

> **Case study 10.4 Case-based consultation involving the review of unit procedures: Jack, 10 years**
>
> From the time Jack arrived in the unit, he would self-harm on a daily basis by eating broken pieces of glass. This behaviour could not be anticipated and raised great anxiety among the staff, resulting in Jack being placed in his room under close supervision. The manager brought this to the attention of the consultant in one of their meetings and in conjunction with the key worker they reviewed the daily records. The resulting formulation was that Jack's behaviour was not indicative of suicidal intent, rather it was functional to remove himself from the other children and to obtain high levels of contact with the staff group.
>
> A care plan for Jack was devised such that his key worker developed structured activities for Jack on a one-to-one basis with staff in the communal areas of the unit. The plan also included a graded introduction of other children into the activities.
>
> With regard to the self–harming behaviour it was agreed that at such times Jack would be placed in his room, and although staff were obliged to provide high levels of checks this was to be done in a pragmatic manner with minimal interactions with Jack.

The care plan enabled Jack to obtain his close positive interactions with staff through appropriate behaviour at times when he was out in the communal areas and conversely to not receive high levels of interaction at times of inappropriate behaviour. This reinforced increases in appropriate positive behaviour and a decrease in inappropriate self-harming behaviour.

Having agreed the care plan, the manager with the key worker then facilitated a team meeting where the care plan was discussed with staff having opportunities to raise any concerns prior to implementation. It was also emphasised that consistency of approach across all staff was critical.

Owing to the high levels of anxiety experienced by the staff, it was agreed that the consultant would be available for telephone consultation in between visits if required. However, this was not taken up and at the next visit it was reported that Jack's self-harming behaviour had stopped within two days of implementing the plan. Although Jack continued to struggle to engage with the other children, he was able to undertake activities in the same room with them.

## Key features arising from the consultant's experience of offering consultation to the young people's secure unit

Offering a mental health provision to a secure unit is difficult without the inclusion of training, direct clinical work and consultation. Consultation can be viewed, in fact, as the overarching framework from which all other work evolves.

Consultation is important both in identifying and enabling, as well as being a valuable link to and from direct clinical work.

- Consultation provides a means of identifying levels of knowledge and skill to facilitate the staff in their direct work with the young people and the development of the unit ethos. Such a process enables the information that already exists about the young person, including mental health assessments, to be collated and guides the work undertaken with the focus on effecting *change* rather than merely managing risk.

- The consultation also enables the identification of specified training fora. This also requires knowledge of the training and previous experience of the members of staff and recognisation that there is likely to be a high level of variability. Links with the social services and Youth Justice Board training departments would be beneficial in this regard.
- It is important to ensure that there is basic training that all members of staff are able to benefit from, including foundation behaviour management principles and parent skills training such as Webster Stratton Incredible Years Training. The key elements to training for staff in mental health in such an environment would be to enable them to understand and facilitate conditions conducive to good mental health and to develop an understanding of attachment, trauma and related interventions.
- Equally, limited direct work helps develop relationships and facilitates the consultation process, as well as providing credibility for the consultant (after all, why should anyone engage in a helping relationship with you in the absence of solid evidence that you know what you are talking about?). Direct clinical work can be utilised in an assessment format or can be seen as a training opportunity in itself, through co-working. It can therefore be useful to be familiar with a range of therapeutic approaches to inform the consultation. Overall, within the context of secure accommodation, cognitive-behaviour interventions have been found to be most effective. As a high proportion of the population has experienced considerable trauma and disrupted attachments, some knowledge and experience of attachment therapy and trauma work are essential, as is a systemic practice to function within the organisational context as well as promote the community, social and family context of the young person. Finally, substance misuse is another common issue facing these young people and relapse prevention and the stages-of-change model are particularly useful approaches.

## Conclusion: consultation as a framework for mental health provision

Consultation offers a significant means of being able to support and facilitate direct work with children by enhancing the skills and confidence of front-line workers. It can also be used to help to develop the context in which staff and children alike are living. Some of the advantages have been discussed in the preceding sections and can be summarised as follows.

---

**Consultation as a framework for mental health provision**

- Develops mutual knowledge and understanding
- Helps identify practitioner levels of knowledge and skill and thereby facilitation of individual and team practice

- Provides a platform for the development of the unit's therapeutic ethos
- Enables training needs to be identified and met
- Improves practice through providing co-working opportunities

The consultant needs to be familiar with relevant areas of work and skilled in their application.

## Systemic perspective

The initial attempts to engage with the unit demonstrate how important it is to hold a systemic perspective. It was particularly important for the consultant to be able to gain an understanding of the history of the unit, its context within the community and other agencies, as well as the hierarchy of formal and informal structures within the unit itself. Critical to this is clarifying who are the key stakeholders and recognising that there might be multiple levels of input required at differing times.

Essential within this is the support and commitment of management, not only to facilitate the development of consultation provision but for management to offer the reliable, predictable and consistent care to staff that they expect staff to provide to the young people.

This further highlights the importance of communication and ensuring that good liaison occurs across staff, professions and agencies as there is a high potential for splitting to occur in such environments.

An awareness of the cultural context is important. Consultation can be used to help facilitate the unit's development of an overarching ethos, preferably a therapeutic milieu model with clear structure, routines and support fora for the staff. This should include specified time for children with regard to education, recreation, individual direct work and group work or discussions. The emphasis is on structure as a basis for security. There is also an important emphasis on each staff member having a clear role and remit and, from a mental health perspective, developing the key worker function. Within this context it is also important for the consultant to maintain a mental health perspective. It is preferable therefore for them to be based within a mental health service and offer an outreach provision into the secure unit, rather than be based within the unit itself.

## Establishing consultation fora: 'if at first you don't succeed . . .'

For the consultant who doesn't give up, the process is a circular one, with each element informing, supporting and driving the next. Where staff are not ready or able to take up the formal consultation forum, the opportunity will inevitably present itself at another point in the cycle. In this unit, it proved to be not the best place to start. When the time is right, there are a number of conditions that will help it to be successful.

- It is important to be familiar with the environment and have the opportunity to meet with all staff and facilitate their collaboration in the service provision by offering their ideas, suggestions and concerns. This will aid ownership and take-up of the service.

- This focus on collaboration extends to the consultation forum itself, in recognising that each participant in the consultation process comes with a range of experience and skills alongside gaps in their knowledge. It is the shared process of understanding that will lead to useful and creative opportunities for work with these young people.
- In the consultation context, as has previously been mentioned, the process can only succeed if the consultee feels safe and clear about the purpose of the forum and there is clarity regarding responsibility of decision making and the recording of information.
- It is also important that the consultation occurs in a regular place and time, provides containment for the staff and models reliability and predictability.
- It is also worth noting that it does take time for staff to become acclimatised to change and to a new service provision. In particular, regular reminders and the physical presence of the consultant can help to facilitate this. Finally, it is beneficial to distinguish between supervision and consultation, in particular emphasising that supervision is through the professional hierarchy and encouraging such a process (the experience of many consultants is that it needs a lot of encouraging).
- Within a secure setting there are structures, procedures and protocols that can support – and be supported by – the consultation process. For example, consultations can be used not only to review initial assessments and help with the care planning, but also to help in the process of planning for discharge.
- As always, regular reviews and evaluation of the provision are essential to enable adjustment. This must include the possibility of not offering consultation, as seen earlier, if workers do not have sufficient levels of skill to make use of it. Under such circumstances, it is important that the consultant uses the experience to highlight what else might be useful at that particular time (e.g. specific training programmes).

## Specific issues relevant to children's secure units

Clearly a key feature of the consultation process will require the consultant to be familiar with the client population in order to be able to help staff to disentangle – and balance – the varying priorities in terms of the children's presenting difficulties and agency requirements. It is important to recognise that mental health priorities may vary from social care and youth justice priorities (*see* Chapter 5) and thought needs to be given to facilitating the staff in being able to consider both and fulfil statutory requirements.

In particular with this population, the discharge process is an area of difficulty as children are reviewed appropriately on a regular basis to see whether they continue to meet criteria. However, if there has been little graded linking with the community, though the child may not meet criteria within the unit there is little information available as to whether they meet criteria when away from the unit.

## Support for the consultant

As with all professional codes of conduct, in the consultant role there is a requirement to recognise the limits of one's abilities, role and remit. Within such contexts it is likely that the consultant will experience strong emotions of feeling overwhelmed or anxious following the sharing of worries by staff or in the face of the overwhelming needs of the unit/young people. It is critical that the consultant has their own supervision to be able to act on the dynamics and to provide focus and containment. Being based away from the unit in a mental health service setting will further enable them to remain objective and focused on mental health issues.

# References

Boswell G (1998) Research-minded practice with young offenders who commit grave crimes. *Probation Journal*.

*Children Act 1989* (c.41). HMSO, London.

*Children and Young Person Act 1933*. HMSO, London.

*Children and Young Person Act 1969*. HMSO, London.

*Crime and Disorder Act 1998*. HMSO, London.

Department for Education and Skills (2003) *National Statistics: children accommodated in secure units. Year ending 31 March 2003: England and Wales*. HMSO, London.

Department of Health (2000) *Adoption: a new approach*. HMSO, London.

Hagell A (2002) *The Mental Health of Young Offenders: bright futures – working with vulnerable young people*. Policy Research Bureau, Mental Health Foundation, London.

Hobbs and Hook Consulting (2001) *Research into Effective Practice with Young People in Secure Facilities*. Report to the Youth Justice Board. Hobbs and Hook Consulting.

Mental Health Foundation (1999) *The Big Picture: promoting children and young people's mental health*. Mental Health Foundation, London.

NACRO (2003) *The Links Between YOTS and Social Services*. NACRO, London.

NACRO (2004) *Youth Crime Briefing: some facts about young people who offend – 2002*. NACRO, London.

National Audit Office (2004) *Youth Offending: the delivery of community and custodial sentences*. National Audit Office, London.

National Health Service/Health Advisory Service (1995) *Child and Adolescent Mental Health Services. Together We Stand: the commissioning role and management of child and adolescent mental health services*. HMSO, London.

*Powers of the Criminal Courts (Sentencing) Act 2000*. HMSO, London.

Richardson J and Joughin C (2000) *The Mental Health Needs of Looked-After Children*. Gaskell, London.

Youth Justice Board (2000) *Secure Facilities Placement Guidance*. April.

Youth Justice Board (2001a) *Research into Effective Practice with Young People in Secure Facilities*. Research note no. 3, April. Youth Justice Board, London.

Youth Justice Board (2001b) *Secure Facilities Placement*. Guidance no. 4, September. Youth Justice Board, London.

Youth Justice Board (2001c) *Risk Factors Associated with Youth Crime and Effective Remedies to Prevent It*. Research note no. 5, November. Youth Justice Board, London.

# Chapter 11

# Teaching consultation skills: the manager as consultant

*Rita Harris*

## Introduction

This chapter describes the process of developing training in applying systemic ideas to the task of management. Within this theoretical model, certain aspects of the role of manager parallel those of the consultant providing consultancy within their own organisation, whether to individuals, groups or to the organisation in its entirety. Consultation is viewed as a process of creating conditions for the consultee to utilise their inner resources and potential. This may involve facilitating awareness of the anxieties that might get in the way of working effectively so as to open up new options (Huffington *et al.* 1997). Although there are, inevitably, aspects of the role of manager that involve issues of responsibility, these aspects should be clear and distinct from the consultative process itself, which rests on the assumption that responsibility for the decisions and their consequences remain with the consultee. This distinction is important, as the process by which one might enable individuals to discover new ways of working is often a consultative one.

The process of developing the training programme described in this chapter also reflects a personal journey from having been a manager within the National Health Service (NHS) to training others in managing processes. For the trainer, as is often the case for a manager, the task is to take a 'metaposition' in relation to those undergoing training. Systemic thinking is a way of enabling people to do just that, by stepping back and observing their own position within the system. By doing so we become aware of the various influences on us, and the ways in which we influence others in the organisation. If the trainer can attend explicitly to their own contribution to the process of learning and the feedback loops this creates, the opportunity presents itself to demonstrate the processes themselves under discussion. The idea of position rather than self is central to systemic thinking in that it enables us to see people occupying many different positions in (many) different contexts. Thus participants are encouraged to observe and reflect on their role and to attempt to stand a little outside the interactions and organisation of which they are a part. In this way they are more likely to be influenced by new ideas and possibilities, i.e. new feedback. The challenge to the trainer in taking such a position also reflects the dilemma faced by participants. These concepts are described in more detail later in the chapter.

In general, people undertake management training wanting to learn how to manage. Often this means to them how to take charge and do it 'properly'. The approach described here is somewhat different to traditional approaches to management and consultancy, i.e. that of expert. Within a systemic framework our expertise lies in an ability to facilitate others to come to a new understanding of the way problems are constructed and maintained in organisations. The training described in this chapter was designed to help effect a shift in thinking about how to manage what is essentially a contextual process – a process of reflection allowing people to think about their actions and what these mean both to themselves and others. This helps them observe their experiences in a way that allows participants to appreciate the contexts in which they are acting and begin to develop new perspectives on these actions. It also gives an opportunity to connect current experiences to others they have had previously and hence generalise from these.

Another key idea that has been useful in developing new thinking and behaviour has been in facilitating participants' awareness of the narratives or stories they have developed about becoming a manager. The ability to accept new ideas can be restricted by not questioning cultural and personally developed ideas that limit choice and the ability to change. By identifying some of these narratives and alternative possibilities, people have found it possible to change the narratives they have about management and themselves within this role and, as a consequence, to act differently.

The course under discussion in this chapter does not claim to teach management: it could be argued that management is not something that can be taught. Rather, the methods described facilitate learning and development in a largely consultative way, encouraging participants to become observers of themselves and others, whilst attending to and being influenced by feedback. This is based on two central ideas. Firstly that systems thinking enables us to understand better the effects of connectedness in organisations and offers us ways of thinking about dilemmas and tensions that arise. Secondly, when people understand and accept how they and others create and maintain ideas about organisations and their problems, they are able to change these understandings and find new ways of behaving.

As a manager is a member of an organisation, their ideas are limited by the feedback received. A consultant may be considered better able to be an observer and have a different – perhaps wider – view and one that might introduce new ideas. This is possible because the consultant is not being organised by the same feedback as are the members of the organisation. Therefore, the consultant and manager both have to work collaboratively in order to arrive at a shared understanding of the difficulties and to generate new ideas. However, the expertise of both consultant and manager in the area being explored is less relevant than the skills of involving others in a collaborative process of exploration. It is important to look for the interactive processes that create meanings about the organisation and relationships within it, and can prevent change from happening. Clearly, the capacity to take a different perspective on presenting problems is more complicated for a manager than a consultant who has been brought in to consult to an organisation. However, no consultant can be neutral and, like the manager, must try to be aware of their particular biases and take responsibility for how they interact with the organisation. The challenge is not to hold on too tightly to one's own views and turn them into 'truths'.

This chapter provides a brief description of the training, the underlying theoretical premises and some of the issues faced by the participants. Through examples, it illustrates some of the ways that those undergoing training put their newly discovered ideas into action. It includes some reflection on the processes and benefits of learning, as experienced by trainees themselves, inevitably raising some organisational dilemmas along the way.

# The training course

The course has been developed and delivered over a number of years by trainers who have extensive experience of managing services in health and education.

Training is delivered in two blocks of three days of (intensive) seminars and workshops separated by a gap of six months. The seminars are designed to provide a theoretical framework within which to reflect upon the processes of management within public sector organisations. Course members develop a systemic framework and understanding of organisations that they can apply to their own work contexts via a mixture of formal teaching and experiential exercises. Throughout the training, participants are encouraged to explore the processes involved in carrying out management tasks, reflecting on their own experiences and common concerns. Central to our thinking is the importance of reflectiveness – the capacity to monitor and reflect on one's own actions and ideas. Participants are offered numerous opportunities to translate theory into practice, the feedback from these experiences enabling them to change the way they understand and approach tasks.

During the six-month course, members complete a project in which they are required to apply the systemic ideas from the course and their reading to a management task they are engaged in. This, plus participation on the course, is something they are required to negotiate with their line manager within their organisation. The course members are each assigned a tutor (from the staff team of four) whom they may consult about their project. There is a day in the middle of the six-month gap when course members meet in small groups with their tutors. These groups offer invaluable peer consultation on the projects. They also often continue beyond the course as peer consultation groups. It is not easy to maintain the position of observer (see below) whilst engaged in the daily task of management and the staff group, and course members, have found a consulting peer group invaluable in managing these processes.

# Basic premises

The basic premises that guided the process of teaching and consultation differ from traditional management, i.e. that difficulties can be solved by the application of good practice, which can be imposed in a linear, often hierarchical way.

## The organisation as an interconnected system

Within systemic thinking, organisations are understood as interconnected systems of relationships that are constituted and regulated by feedback in a recursive pattern. Change in one relationship in a system changes all others. Therefore one must always consider the effect of any change on other relationships. For example, a number of managers find themselves in newly appointed roles, often within services where they were previously working in a different role. They often have the experience of struggling to establish a role and mandate for themselves. Case study 11.1 illustrates how a course participant used such a dilemma to rethink his position.

---

**Case study 11.1**

One educational psychologist had been recently appointed as a specialist educational psychologist to promote inclusion across a local education authority (LEA). During the course of training, he shifted his thinking from seeing those outside the Educational Psychology Service (EPS) as being resistant and needing managing to an idea that the issue he was seeking to address was part of a larger process. He concluded that being appointed to an LEA-wide brief by one professional grouping without reference to any other group reflected issues about how that professional group related to the LEA. He became interested in who the stakeholders were, the organisational culture and beliefs (see below) in relation to inclusion and the recursive interactions within and between different systems.

---

Systemic theory is not an explanatory theory; rather it is a framework for observing and understanding the world in terms of the connections among its parts. Our expertise lies in an ability to facilitate others to come to a new understanding of the way problems are constructed and maintained.

## The observer as part of the process

Central to this way of thinking about organisations is that no one is removed from the feedback loops that connect all parts of the organisation. The observer is considered to be part of the process (Von Foerster 1981), with a system being defined by the position of the observer and the meaning attached to such observing. What we choose to observe, the questions we ask, the feedback we attend to and the meaning we ascribe to it are influenced by our assumptions and beliefs (see below). It is therefore a central aim of the trainers to enable managers to observe the levels of meaning they are influenced by and why these lead to particular interpretations and consequent behaviour. By being supported in taking this 'observer' position, course members are able to become aware of various influences on themselves and the ways in which they, in turn, influence others. This new awareness often results in their developing new ways of understanding situations and behaving differently, resulting in new interactions and feedback loops.

This relates to the concept of *reflexivity*, which is central in systemic thinking. We are reminded that we are both autonomous individuals on the one hand and participants of interaction processes on the other. Taking a reflexive position helps us observe ourselves and take responsibility for our part in the process.

## Feedback

It is feedback that connects all parts of the system, and demonstrates the interdependence of relationships. Feedback over time creates patterns through which events and behaviour acquire meaning. In this way feedback may be seen as the lifeblood of a system, the means by which information is exchanged. We all act on the basis of ideas about what is appropriate/valuable/rewarding in any given context. These ideas are based on the feedback we receive and in turn influence how we understand and think about the behaviour of others and ourselves.

In organisations communication difficulties can arise from communication practices that preclude debate and conflict about values. For feedback to be useful, differences between people and points of view need to be seen as a resource and not a threat, in order to create new ideas. In the example below new feedback was made possible partly by recognising the importance of the responsible individuals to come together in a way that created a new context for differences to be discussed. In this way, new and unexpected feedback emerged.

---

**Case study 11.2**

Two course members from the same service joined one another to try to find ways of functioning in their new management roles. The context was a service in turmoil, understaffed teams and difficulties in recruiting to an organisation that was being completely reorganised. What emerged from a long and well-structured consultation process, sanctioned and welcomed by the two most influential people in the organisation, as part of the course work, were profound differences in their overall vision for the service and ways of communicating to one another and the organisation generally. By using the vehicle of feedback from the consultation process, different options for how the service might be delivered, and some of the dilemmas each of these represented, emerged and a competitive deadlock was made apparent without being named as such. For these course members the importance of feedback helped them think about how the problems had occurred rather than why.

---

## Context

Understanding an organisation as a system is also about understanding the many contexts and meanings people use to govern their behaviour. Systems exist for a purpose and this creates the context, i.e. gives meaning to the activity that takes place. An important aim of the training is therefore to enable people to observe the levels of meaning they are influenced by and, in turn, to be able to facilitate this in others. It is assumed that by developing an understanding of the meaning and values of an organisation, we begin to develop an understanding of its culture.

A theme that came through all the projects was the usefulness of widening a 'problematic' context via mapping the key players in the system and asking systemic questions (Campbell *et al.* 1994). This refers to some composite of the discourses and activities within an organisation that represents it. Problems can arise when certain experiences are selected over others and become privileged in the organisation. When this happens people begin to attribute meanings to their actions on the basis of the way behaviour fits into pre-existing concepts. The challenge, as illustrated in Case study 11.3 below, is to discover creative, liberating conversations that enable us to create new meanings and overcome apparent obstacles.

---

**Case study 11.3**

A newly appointed manager felt criticised and something of a failure in not being able to ensure her service responded to a senior manager's directions to collate monthly activity data. By meeting the information officer, whose task it was to collate information across the trust, she discovered how poorly the activity criteria fitted her service and the important way in which these data were being used to represent the service. She explored the meaning of auditing and evaluating services for the team, herself and trust managers. This resulted in a shift in her and the team's position from seeing data collection as meaningless to a tool that could communicate more clearly to others what the service provided. The team, with the help of the information officer, explored how to feedback information more helpfully and participate in the development of a new database. Feedback from the information officer was also very positive. She had previously felt disconnected from the services she was working with and often felt regarded with suspicion and dislike.

---

Campbell (2000) discusses the usefulness of metaphor to a consultant interested in change. He sees its value in being 'unfamiliar' and not yet absorbed into 'meaningful language'. In Campbell's view, 'Fitting into the familiar is also constraining the participants to only certain meanings which have already been agreed, whereas metaphor may be used in conversation to introduce a difference to the conventional meaning of the words being used.'

An appreciation that our thinking about organisations is often reflected as metaphorical concepts can help us become aware that this is not a 'truth', but a *construction* that may privilege or highlight certain ideas at certain times.

---

**Case study 11.4**

One course participant became interested in the idea of metaphors to work with organisations. As someone who had not been keen to move into a management role, he used a metaphor to maintain a degree of neutrality in exploring his new role and the organisation. He chose that of an art student exploring an idea. He began by keeping a systemic sketchbook of situations and issues he encountered. This was designed to capture quickly and schematically incidents that caught his interest during the day. Inevitably he took some of these fragments home and worked on them. Taking the role of an artist encouraged this course member to work systemically – observe closely; find ways to elaborate by seeking more information; change the focus from close-up portraits to broader landscapes. In his view the idea of a sketch encouraged a sense that individual perceptions of a situation are partial, incomplete, subject to later revision and may display some artistic licence. When he shared these ideas with others in his service this generated feedback that was unexpected. People were able to connect and relate to how he might develop his role as a manager and the anxieties he initially had about the role. In this example one can see how this stance enabled this participant to formulate hypotheses (hunches) about what was happening. Hypotheses here are regarded not in terms of ultimate truth or falseness but in terms of how helpful they were in facilitating his understanding of the situation and facilitating some positive change (Palazzoli *et al.* 1980). Through this process of hypothesising he was able to punctuate events in new ways, allowing new ideas to emerge (Palazzoli *et al.* 1978).

## Organisational culture and constructed realities

Social constructionism (Burr 1995; Campbell 2002) has been helpful in focusing on how people work together to construct the realities they live in. Social constructionism emphasises the centrality of relationships. We only become people through being involved in a central world of meanings through our interactions with others. It suggests that our social world is actively created by interactions within and between groups of people in society. What is created is a set of ideas or shared beliefs that lead to various practices and behaviours. It acknowledges that there are social realities, dominant beliefs and ways of thinking about the world. For further reading on the subject, see Burr (1995). Here social discourse and social practices are seen as the building blocks that enable us to make sense of our lives.

The theory invites us to consider what are the *dominant* – i.e. those given privilege – and the *submerged* – i.e. not privileged – discourses in various policies, meetings and conversations. So participants are encouraged to be interested in what can and cannot be said and the meaning and power of these conversations for the organisation and roles within it. This enables course members to explore their organisational cultures, i.e. shared meanings based on shared assumptions and beliefs that operate to define the system. These basic ideas and assumptions guide behaviour. The current training programme has devised a number of exercises with the aim of helping explore the dominant and marginalised discourses in organisations. The focus is on listening carefully to the language used, the values embedded within it, and what alternatives there might be and at what cost.

Questions have included:

- What are the main beliefs that govern your organisation?
- Who holds them?
- What is the language used to express those beliefs?

- Identify some dominant and marginalised discourses.
- Whose voices get heard?

What many participants have experienced is that proposed organisational changes have challenged theirs and others' narratives, e.g. about what they value about their work or how they feel valued at work. An example of an exercise you might like to try for yourself is appended at the end of this chapter.

Course members have found it extremely helpful to explore situations where there appears to be a mismatch between what an individual perceives to be of value and that of the organisation as a whole.

## Fit

People are in a position of trying to balance their individual needs, ideas and beliefs with those of the group and the wider context. We work for a variety of reasons: income, personal satisfaction, status, etc. Here there is an assumption that when personal gains are met through work, the employee will be satisfied and continue to work for the good of the organisation. However, when the organisational task is unsatisfying or in conflict with individual needs, people may become less motivated to co-operate in this. Systemic thinkers are always interested in problems of 'fit' between the parts of an organisation and the parts of the whole. However, whilst the components of the system must fit, there must also be sufficient difference and diversity among the parts for each to be defined and for creativity to be possible. A system needs to be flexible and to adjust to new feedback. One of the most effective ways we found in enabling course members to explore problems of fit that often resulted in a sense of feeling 'stuck' was to examine the potential losses and gains inherent in change and the dilemmas thrown up by this.

## Change and stability: losses and gains

There is an assumption in systemic thinking that organisations need to balance change with stability. Here systems acquire a stability that people can recognise and build on, and when roles and relationships are seen as changing too much, individuals may feel as though their connection to a stable organisation is threatened. It is proposed that organisational change brings possible losses and gains and that one needs to arrive at an understanding of what these mean to individuals and the ways in which these perspectives become incorporated into the culture of an organisation.

What many course members experienced was that as the pace of change increased, the possible gains and losses came into sharper focus, leading to more self-protective behaviour on behalf of their team members. Whilst ostensibly agreeing to the principles, one service had a very low uptake of new pro formas designed to support the (new) consultative approaches to case-work and provide data on effectiveness of interventions. This low uptake was despite a great deal of team time having gone into agreeing to work in this way and designing the form together. This course member held an open forum in which the team could reflect on the losses and gains implied by the changes for them, and on people's ideas about how to manage the implications of change. By focusing on issues of personal investment and security, rather than the details of the forms, this course member was able to help manage some of the processes.

A common finding in much of the work course members did was that proposed changes and service developments were being managed with consensus being an implicit and central objective. The process seemed to often avoid open discussion of some of the key dilemmas for individuals and groups that change poses. There was often a poor correspondence between consensual language used to describe and reflect upon service changes and the meanings attached to that language. Indeed, on closer examination one often found disparity about the meaning of core tasks and a lack of clarity about boundaries between systems and what each offers. This was demonstrated in Case study 11.1, when the new senior educational psychologist was appointed to promote inclusion across an LEA. He explored what individuals and services meant by inclusion, their views of its usefulness, their views of his role and their roles, and the relationships between these. It has been very helpful to encourage course members to take their time in mapping and exploring some of the dilemmas and the meanings of those they have faced. This has often resulted in open discussion of some of the dilemmas faced by individuals and organisations and greater clarity about roles.

## Conclusions

Within this framework, organisational consultants and managers are shifting from traditional ways of thinking about organisations. The first is from ideas of cause and effect, blame and dysfunction to the idea of interconnected events and behaviours resulting from beliefs, which link different parts of the system. Feedback from these events either confirms or challenges those beliefs. There is also a shift from being an expert to an explorer and co-creator. Participants learn the value of curiosity and how to facilitate this in others in order to develop a more reflective observer position (Cecchin 1987).

Course participants reported valuing the experience of being listened to and given space to reflect on their assumptions, beliefs and behaviour. They saw this as an important part of the process of developing new roles and ways of working. They also highlighted the importance of role definition and clarity and a greater awareness of the complexity of organisational processes. Participants became increasingly aware of how organisational processes, e.g. overt versus covert dialogues, needed managing in order to achieve this. This is referring to the importance of trying to understand the meanings attached to these and what perceived losses and dilemmas are thrown up in the process.

For most, organisational change meant developing an understanding of its culture and finding ways of creating new conversations in which all views of all members of the organisation can find a 'voice', whether dominant or marginalised. In this way the dilemmas faced can be opened up for examination and new possibilities emerge.

Probably the most important aspect of learning seems to be the development of a greater capacity for self-reflection. This enables not only the individual to become more self-observant but also to develop this skill in others. This process is key in the development of new narratives about themselves as managers of processes. All felt that the time spent doing so was well invested but often felt unable to maintain this position once back at work. In order to continue in this process many have continued to meet as consulting pairs or groups.

Many felt clearer about their role in their organisation, which often brought with it fewer feelings of blame and anxiety about responsibility. This seemed to be facilitated by a greater awareness of the interconnectedness of organisations and an appreciation of the importance of wider contexts. Similarly, there was an appreciation of the complexity of organisations and how fruitless time spent on detail can be without an understanding of the context and therefore the meaning attached to any action or behaviour. These became more important to course members than the need to be able to give the best 'top down' directions, which for those of us running the course was considered to be a positive outcome from this form of consultation.

Whether acting as an outside consultant or manager, all found it challenging to explore new ideas rather than propose solutions, particularly when under pressure to do so without support and supervision. Many who completed the course have developed peer networks that support and challenge one another's ideas.

## Benefits of training

Feedback from course participants has highlighted a number of benefits, which are summarised in Box 11.1. This is a brief course that fits into busy work schedules yet one in which participants experienced quite dramatic outcomes for their role as managers. Firstly, they identified an enhanced capacity to plan strategically and take into account the full organisational context in which they work. Secondly, they have much reduced personal anxiety about their responsibility for every small problematic event. Thirdly, they make more sense of the emotional environment and its impact upon the processes of achieving outcomes.

During the course participants are continually asked to apply the ideas developed to their work context, which provides immediate feedback demonstrating both the usefulness and relevance of the ideas to a number of contexts. It is difficult to become a systemic manager. The demands, which predominate in any management role, tend to be reactive and premised on cause and effect thinking, often with no time to pause and reflect. This framework provides opportunities to reflect, to observe and to consult with others who share similar challenges. Having completed this course, participants have explored and developed new ways of working within their organisations. Applications and projects require support from line managers and a statement of what they hope the course will offer this staff member. In this way we hope to introduce ideas of connection and feedback from the outset.

# Exercise

---

**Narratives about management**

1 What in your view is the purpose of management?
2 What do you think makes a good manager? (How would you know?)
3 What is your management style?
4 How would you describe your manager?
5 What would you like to be different about your current managerial arrangements? (What stops this? What would facilitate it?)
6 What are the beliefs/rules about management in your organisation?

---

**Box 11.1 Summary of the benefits of training**

- Cost-effective in terms of the brief investment of time
- Managers who feel less anxious and more curious about potential organisational changes
- Tasks are applied to participants' work context – immediate feedback/return
- Generalisable to any context
- Self-reflection is useful in a range of settings/tasks
- Possibilities of developing an internal consultant to the organisation
- Approach to organisational change may become more thoughtful and potentially slower but more effective

# References

Burr V (1995) *An Introduction to Social Constructionism.* Routledge, London.

Campbell D (2000) *The Socially Constructed Organisation.* Karnac Books, London.

Campbell D, Coldicott T and Kinsella K (1994) *Systemic Work With Organisations.* Karnac Books, London.

Cecchin G (1987) Hypothesizing, circularity and neutrality revisited: an invitation to curiosity. *Family Process.* **26**: 405–13.

Huffington C, Cole C and Brunning H (1997) *A Manual of Organizational Development.* Karnac Books, London.

Palazzoli MS, Boscolo L, Cecchin G *et al.* (1980) Hypothesizing–circularity–neutrality: three guidelines for the conductor of the session. *Family Process.* **19** (1): 3–12.

Palazzoli MS, Cecchin G, Prata G *et al.* (1978) *Paradox and Counter-Paradox: a new model in the therapy of family in schizophrenic transaction.* Jason Aronson, New York.

Von Foerster H (1981) *Observing Systems.* Intersystems Publications, Seaside, CA.

# Chapter 12

# The last word . . . consultation with service users

*Donna Wedgbury, Machita Denny, Kate Stokes, Thelma Barlow, Caitlyn Staples and Emma Probert with Angela Southall*

The last word on consultation surely belongs with service users themselves. In this chapter, service users describe their experiences of consulting to services and individuals through organised user groups, in an advisory role or during the course of their own or their children's involvement with a service. All have important stories to tell.

The current national emphasis on user involvement in services has led to a number of service-led schemes to place users at the centre of healthcare developments. Such schemes are not the business of this chapter. Rather, its focus is on the *experiences* of users who have become involved in service development and delivery in an advisory or consultative role. Many such experiences are user-led. In this chapter, service users contribute to a picture of user involvement and consultation. They include foster carers, organisers of a support group for parents of children with autism, carers who have shared the therapeutic journey with their children, a parent who has a formal advisory role with an NHS trust and young people who have themselves experienced mental health problems and been users of mental health services. It can only be a snapshot of user involvement but it is a fascinating and important one.

The chapter begins with an account by Donna Wedgbury of her experiences as an 'Associate Director' service user in a mental health trust and moves on from this to explore other service users' experiences.

## How Associate Directors can contribute to services

Donna is an Associate Director with South Staffordshire Healthcare NHS Trust. She was appointed with five other service users as part of a drive towards greater user involvement, following the Trust's successful bid for funding from the Workforce Development Confederation. The Associate Director posts are salaried and they have an office at Trust Headquarters, which gives them easy access to the Chief Executive and Chair.

The Associates have particular areas of interest and experience, although they have a free reign to get involved in any aspect they wish. Donna's experiences as a mother of a little boy with cerebral palsy mean that her interests lie firmly in the area of children's services. Like the other Associates, Donna finds herself doing far more than her allotted one day a week.

The project so far seems to have been effective. A recent six-month evaluation finds that 'associates have become involved at every level of the organisation in a wide range of geographical locations and service areas' (Green 2004).

Donna's experiences of the project have also been positive. She admits that, to begin with, there were concerns. 'We all asked ourselves, is this tokenism? But the answer has to be "no": we are having a real impact. People are asking for our views and listening to them.' The evaluation document supports this view:

> Several of the Associates commented on initial concern that they might lose their service user focus and not be able to speak out on behalf of those they were appointed to represent. At the present stage, they do not report feeling compromised by being Trust employees. After six months, nearly all are reporting increased confidence and authority in this role and they have clearly earned wide respect and recognition in the organisation. The value of this in promoting working partnerships with service users and carers should not be underestimated.
>
> (Green 2004)

The Associates, like Donna, are in a unique position, giving a voice to service users and providers and consulting at a senior management level in the Trust. Donna has first-hand experience of what can happen as a result:

> I met with some parents of children with disabilities in Lichfield, where they are looking towards having a new children's centre. Until they get the centre, there are lots of gaps in services. We were able to set up a new toddlers' group with specialist health visitors and physiotherapists. We found that many people were willing to give time voluntarily, including a nursery nurse. The Child Health Director made funding available for the hire of a hall for one afternoon a week. All this came from one meeting with parents!

Another example Donna gives is of training by speech and language therapists to parents of children with autism spectrum disorder (ASD), so that they can make the most of the school-based sessions their children have. This was delivered during the summer holidays and also grew out of a stance of taking parents seriously as consultants and, in turn, being able to act as a consultant to others.

These are examples of the real value of engaging service users as consultants. They also suggest, strongly, that the Associates take their roles very seriously. Green (2004) cites one of the Associates in her evaluation:

> When I have attended meetings outside the Trust and informed other carers and professionals about the scheme, there have been two reactions. One is that people have been impressed with the Trust for taking this step, followed by 'Isn't this just a tick-box scheme?' My response is that it could have been but we simply aren't tick-box people.

### What more can Associate Directors do?

Donna is keen to involve parents and carers more in direct service provision, both in terms of offering support to others and acting as advocates. She feels parent and carer representatives have a lot to offer. In particular, she would like to see service users providing more feedback on services and in key customer service roles where they can offer training to professionals. Service users, she says, can tell us the things we don't always want to hear. As Donna puts it, 'It is the little things that make the difference.'

It looks as though the new Associate Director posts are, indeed, starting to make a difference:

> There are signs that the Associate Directors are having a considerable impact and increasing the momentum of a major cultural shift towards the development of more meaningful partnerships in healthcare between service users and providers.
>
> (Green 2004)

For Donna, this is not entirely new. Through her son, Harvey, she has often found herself playing a key role in giving a voice to parents' concerns, as well as sharing her knowledge and experience with service providers. Her advice is twofold: for service users to get involved and make themselves heard and, as for providers, we should all take note: 'Service users are the greatest resource you have.'

The following section describes how a group of parents and carers of children with ASD organise themselves to offer support to each other and take on a growing advisory role within the organisation.

## The Jigsaw Group

Machita Denny is secretary of the Jigsaw Group, a voluntary user support group with a difference. The group was established in 2001, initially under the auspices of two very dedicated specialists. Over time, the parents themselves began to take responsibility for the group and the professionals took a back-seat advisory role. Today, the group is well established as a parents' group. The first annual general meeting has taken place and the group has achieved charitable status. They produce their own leaflets and newsletter and hold regular meetings with guest speakers, in order to help increase group members' own knowledge about ASD and the myriad of services that are out there. They also organise training, social events for the children and have recently set up a youth club for teenagers who are on the autism spectrum. The group has proved to be a powerful lobbying force and has established itself within the Health Trust. Like Donna and the other Associate Directors, the Jigsaw Group has been given an office at Trust Headquarters and the Chief Executive has agreed to cover some of their costs, including mileage to attend meetings. Machita and her colleague, Janette Talbot, chair of the group, attend the Trust's Service Users Sub-Committee.

For Machita, the group serves many functions, not least the opportunity to talk to other parents and carers in similar circumstances. She finds that service users often worry about giving their views. A common concern is that speaking out might affect the treatment they get. The group helps parents to discover that their opinions can be not only heard but valued and acted upon. Machita is aware that people need support to develop the confidence to have a voice.

Parents of children with autism know all too well that there is going to be no 'quick-fix' solution to their problems. For them, the longer-term view is important. As Machita says, 'You can only see the professionals for a short amount of time and then you're on your own.'

Fortunately, Machita, Janette and the rest of the group have been able to advise on service provision and on what works for them, as well as what they need in terms of ongoing support. They feel their views have always been taken seriously. For their part, they feel they have a valuable contribution to make:

> We have had experiences of services; we can feed back from our point of view. The organisation has a much better idea of what we need, not just what they think we need.

There is recognition among the group that it is important to have service options from which to choose. Each child, young person and family is different and it follows that some things will work better for them than others. Perhaps one of the strongest messages from the group concerns partnership working and integration of services. At the moment, it can be difficult to get a co-ordinated response from health, education and social services. For Machita and the others in the group, this is a challenge. She says, 'We are working and doing our utmost for these children . . . we want you [professionals] to work together.'

Machita's experiences of user involvement have helped her in a number of ways she would not have anticipated:

> . . . it puts you on a different plane of communication with the professionals – you are part of the team. You feel more involved and valued. This all helps with your own feelings of being able to help your child.

This empowerment is important. As she says, 'There is nothing worse than feeling out of control with your own situation.' Speaking to Machita, her enthusiasm is obvious, as is the feeling that the Jigsaw Group is going to go from strength to strength. As she puts it, 'There is more to do: it's just a beginning but it's a good beginning.'

## Cannock Chase Young People's Group

Like many child and adolescent mental health services (CAMHS), Cannock Chase has been actively seeking ways to involve young people in decision making about services for several years. As part of this initiative, two groups of young people made very different contributions to an interagency county conference on child and adolescent mental health. One group did this by attending a weekend film-making workshop, in which they developed ideas for their own short films. With the help of a student film crew, each young person made their own film, from start to finish, taking their completed films home with them at the end of the weekend. The films were shown at the conference as a way of helping the conference audience understand better the experiences of young people who use mental health services. They had an enormous impact.

The second group of young people formed their own 'focus group', attending the conference and providing 'live' feedback to the conference audience on what they were hearing. These young people had follow-up meetings at CAMHS to further advise on services. Some of their views are given below.

## Experiencing and contributing to a conference

All of the young people who participated in the conference found it a helpful and positive experience to meet others who had been users of CAMHS. On the day of the conference, they found themselves in a central role and rose to the occasion quite magnificently. They would later recall it as exciting, valuable and a 'once in a lifetime opportunity'.

The young people were able to raise awareness and understanding among those adults who were present, many of whom were very senior in their respective organisations but who nevertheless felt they learned a great deal from the youngsters themselves:

> I really enjoyed the conference that we did. I found it a learning experience and I liked the fact that there were other people, not necessary exactly in the position I was in but in a similar position. You were not there by yourself and it wasn't just people being paid to help you . . . We talked about our experiences, like how we found CAMHS useful, and how we would like to see it improved and what we thought would help other people.

The young people appreciated having their views listened to and finding themselves in the unusual position of having adult service providers ask for their feedback on services and, clearly, wanting to learn from them.

Without a doubt, there is a lot to learn.

## On advising services

Young CAMHS users feel, quite rightly, that they have a lot to offer in terms of advising about services. After all, they have experienced services at first hand:

> It sounds selfish but if you are here to help us then for you to run smoothly you need to know what we want. There is no point in providing a service that no one has a need for; it's a waste of your time and a waste of our time.

Another focus group member commented that services needed to know 'definitely' what young people want: that practitioners, providers and service users should be 'like an interactive team – you and us.' She went on to say, 'That makes sense. Then it's beneficial for you, the organisation and ourselves.'

The young people agreed that in order to be a mutually useful process, consultation with service users has to have as its basis the relationship between service users and providers. The service user needs to know about the service. They were therefore not keen on the kind of 'tick-box' satisfaction survey that often manifests as user involvement. For them, involvement had to be fairly substantial to be meaningful. As one young person said, 'I don't think you can ask people who have only been a couple of times, unless they know everything that is available to them.'

Another focus group member put it this way:

> . . . they can say, 'I've been twice, I've talked to somebody about it, I am still working through my problems but what else is there . . .' If they don't know they can't say, 'Well actually I would prefer it if I could talk to you at home or I could talk to you at school or I could have your mobile number to speak to you; you know what? I am in crisis right now . . .'

There was a feeling that other service users benefit from the hindsight of those who have experienced the process. However, there was also a view that it was *concurrent* involvement that was most helpful to individual young people themselves. Once having left the service, it was too late to really feel the benefit of any involvement: '. . . to help themselves, it needs to be while they are still with you'.

There were other benefits too, one of which was highlighted as 'closure':

> It gave me closure, in a way, and I could recap on it without starting to stress about it or worry about it. I have been able to . . . put things in a box, review: that happens and that's okay. I can move on. Like, it's part of me but it's not everything.

### Location, location, location

The drive towards community services and, in particular, towards school-based services has been given added impetus by Margaret Hodge's support for the 'open school' philosophy (Clarke *et al.* 2003). This has led to many more partnerships between community CAMHS teams and local schools. In Cannock Chase, the Young People's Group has helped us to think about this and other important issues relating to service delivery, such as where services are located. Interestingly, our service users don't always say what we might expect! For example, service accessibility is far more complicated than making services available in schools or 'shop front' locations. Much of what we might assume is advantageous to young people is felt by them to be fraught with potential difficulties. One focus group member made the following comment about the availability of counselling in school in a not-so-ideal world:

> If it was in school or somewhere more familiar to the people, it would be harder for people to open up because there could be people that they know and know very well and it could cause problems. But in an ideal world that would help because they would be more familiar and it would be easier to set up.

Similarly, when adult service providers talk about accessibility, they often mean that services should be located in a number of neighbourhoods, rather than at a central base which might be a bus ride away. Not always so, say the young people themselves:

> I think if it was any more local to my area, I would have found it a lot more difficult because of people I know. I didn't fit in, anyway – I didn't go to the local school, I lost my dad when I was 10. I was completely isolated from my mates, that's why I changed schools and I'm just so glad that [the service] was away from that. If I saw somebody it would be like, 'Oh yeah, I'm just in Cannock and going to "Greggs".'

When the idea of a 'drop-in' was mooted, there were equally surprising responses. One young person suggested that such a facility would have made it more difficult for her to access help: 'I would prefer it [now], but actually getting me there – I don't think I would have been strong enough to make the first move to go, to know what I needed, to walk into somewhere.' It is difficult for young people to have the kind of information and knowledge of services they need to know that they are safe and staff are approachable and supportive. Young people tell us they are often completely unaware of services before they find themselves on the receiving end of them. Many of them also tell us that, had they had that understanding, they would have had more confidence in accessing help. They would also have sought help sooner.

A number of community CAMHS teams have addressed some of these issues by having young service users consult to them about their information needs and, sometimes, supporting young people to themselves produce publicity and information material. In Cannock Chase, young people who work with us in the local schools as peer mentors have helped set up their own website.

## What more can young people tell us about services?

The young people who use our services in Cannock Chase have helped us shape up many of our ideas about what we do. They are constantly helping us to think about the future and develop ideas about community services that might be able to keep some of the best features of traditional clinic bases whilst losing the worst. Future resources might, it seems, be multi-service centres for young people, having some features in common with youth groups and where service users might also go to socialise. Most of our service users are keen on the 'one-stop shop' idea, where a number of services come together in a single building. At the moment they tell us services are fragmented:

> I don't expect one person to know everything about it.  But . . . then when my dad died, me and my mum got a pension as long as I was in full-time education because my dad was retired. And then . . . I go and see my Connexions officer, and he says, 'Have a year out if you don't know what to do.' And I think, 'Hold on, I can't have a year out because I lose my income if I do that!' He doesn't quite get it; it is not an option to do a year out.  You don't feel you are getting proper advice because they don't know your situation. There is no set route for every single person to go. It's so difficult and so complicated to have all these things in different places.

Just as Donna suggested earlier, young people who use our services see themselves as able to provide much more, in terms of customer services. They can speak from experience and with authority about the services they have used. Many of them do this already, informally, reassuring friends about what is going to happen to them and, sometimes, even explaining to them how to get a referral to their community CAMHS team, some even accompanying them to appointments. As one service user put it, 'I said go and see your doctor for referral to CAMHS. It will take you like a while to get used to it and to get relaxed into it, but being able talk it through without any repercussions, that is the main thing, the security of it. You can say anything you like and nothing is going to happen to you.'

In the end, they acknowledge the important relationship between every therapeutic encounter and the growth and development of the service. Their instinctive awareness of this reflexivity is impressive:

> . . . but it's like: 'I went through that.' Other people are going to go through that and because you know I have gone through it and you have helped me through, you know that's what's going to happen to someone else and you go, 'Okay, well they might feel like this . . . we did it a little bit wrong or we did it bang on. Maybe that's what this persons needs.' So you are more in tune with the next person.

## How foster carers contribute to what we know about looked-after children and how we organise services

Kate Stokes and Thelma Barlow are both 'level four' carers who have, between them, 25 years of experience of fostering young people who have been sexually abused and who have very complex needs.

They are both members of the Carers' Advisory Group of SUSTAIN, a specialist health and social care partnership service in Staffordshire for looked-after young people and their carers. They are involved with a number of different aspects of the service development and delivery, including the following:

- regular meetings with the service co-ordinator to contribute to service development
- representation on the interagency partnership group that oversees the work of the service
- participating in interviews for new therapy staff
- contributing to service promotion through such things as open days.

As a result of their involvement in the Carers' Advisory Group, Kate and Thelma feel they have been able to have an impact on how things have developed. Kate describes their role as being, in part, 'the listening voice for the other carers' and how carers are able to say things to her and to Thelma that they feel unable to say to other professionals. She concludes emphatically, 'And then something is done about it!'

There are other ways, too, that foster carers have an impact on services, many of which are integral to caring. In all sorts of ways, Kate and Thelma have been consulting to professionals for years. For instance, Kate describes fostering teenagers 'when no one else would'. As a result both Thelma and Kate feel that they have had an important role in helping others understand the needs of the children they care for. As Kate says, 'The foster carers live with the child. They know the child . . . we have to be able to advise on the child's needs.'

Thelma feels that more notice of service users has been taken recently, qualifying this by adding, modestly, 'but perhaps I have got more confident in expressing my opinions.' Thelma went on to describe her role in raising awareness and understanding of one of the boys she looked after:

> He came to us, aged 16, from another placement in his home town. He had been looked after since he was 14. We were told that he had a mild learning disability. This child had been sexually abused at the age of nine by a male neighbour. His parents later split up and his mother moved out of the family home. He had a lot of anger towards women and girls and this was something I had to monitor for safe caring.
>
> I did an assessment over three months and, when it was completed, it seemed clear that he had all the signs of autism spectrum disorder. He had some learning difficulties, obsessive insistence on routines and sameness, self-isolation, poor motor control, lack of social awareness and problems with communication and understanding.
>
> I worked with his social worker and leaving care advisor, giving them the assessment of his needs. A report of his behaviour and understanding of social relationships was also submitted to help raise awareness in other agencies that would be supporting him towards independence.

In addition to raising awareness and helping others understand children's needs, foster carers have an important role in shaping up views of professionals regarding the placement of additional children and the idea of 'fit' with those already in placement. Kate describes one of her girls who was displaying very disturbed behaviour, soiling, smearing and wetting, and how she had to turn down a third placement at that time in order to focus her energies on the needs of the children she already had. She says, 'I couldn't take another child because I would have been failing the other two.' Kate's views were taken on board:

> One of the four girls I was looking after at the time was 13 years old but had a developmental age of about eight years. She had learning disabilities and attended a special school. Her behaviour was very disruptive and attention-seeking. She had a tendency to self-harm and would scratch and cut herself and put sharp objects in her ears. She also soiled and smeared. She was very destructive, damaging and defacing her own belongings, as well as those of others. She also had a problem with stealing and lying and would sometimes engage in quite bizarre behaviour, for example licking windows and making strange noises over and over again.
>
> I had meetings with a therapist from SUSTAIN to help make sense of what her behaviours were telling us. I managed her difficult be- haviours with some tried and tested methods I had used over many

years* and supported this with a chart. After one year, the soiling and smearing had stopped and her general behaviour had improved. She was calmer. Although on occasion she still lied, she would own up to it. The same progress was made with her stealing.

Kate feels that in the past it might have been difficult to have such messages heard. Nowadays, there is much more of an acknowledgement that foster carers help link workers and social workers to understand the problems that young people have and to think through difficult placement issues:

> I had two sisters aged 13 and 14. Both girls had been sexually abused by their stepfather from the age of ten years. The older girl became pregnant as a result of this and had a termination. Neither of the girls attended school when they came to me. Both girls displayed extremely challenging, controlling, aggressive behaviour most of the time. Occasionally excessive weeping took place and the girls would sit on the sitting-room floor, arms around each other, weeping and rocking together. This could continue for up to an hour. They could never say why this happened. Both girls returned to full-time education and did well in their GCSEs. The older sister went on to college. At 18 years she began living independently in her own flat. Two years on, she returned to college and still attends. The younger sister became pregnant by her boyfriend at 17 years and moved on to live independently, when she was 18 and a half, in her own flat with the baby's father.

Kate provided a loving home to all three of these girls at the same time, together with another 17-year-old, who moved into independent living at the age of 19.

## Moving towards independence

Thelma talked about the needs of one of her boys, now 20, who has experienced numerous changes in the professionals he has to relate to. He has lived with Thelma and her husband, Ian, for four years and Thelma has been attending therapy with him. When independent living was mooted, Thelma and Ian felt that this young man was not ready. Thelma took the decision to seek the help of the Assistant Director of Social Services himself, 'because this young person didn't fit in any of the boxes'.

> He came to us from another placement where he had been for a year. It was a month before his 16th birthday. He showed all the signs of depression and had made an attempt on his life before he had been removed from home. There were clear signs of developmental delay. He looked about 12 and did not start puberty until he was nearly 17. The history was that he and his elder brother had been sexually abused by their father and groomed for prostitution. He displayed sexualised

---

* Over the years, Kate has often found herself using 'the sandwich technique' when she has a problematic issue to discuss with one of her young people. In essence, this is a 'praise–discuss the problem–praise' formula. We are all indebted to Kate's father, Mr Benjamin George Smart, for teaching her this, as well as how to give a lot of love.

behaviour, low self-esteem, overcompliance, withdrawal and hyper-vigilance. His behaviour became erratic when he was stressed. There were concerns that this boy's abuse continued for some months after the start of the placement with me. Despite everybody's best efforts, he managed to meet his father on a number of occasions and would return bruised and with evidence of sexual activity.

Through the help of SUSTAIN and the therapeutic care that was in place he was able to pull himself away from prostitution. This was at a personal cost to himself as he was threatened and assaulted.

We supported him through these bad times and, at his own pace, encouraged him to join a football team to encourage his confidence in being with 'safe' males. Later, my son got him a job at a fast food outlet where he began to build up his confidence with the general public. His health was up and down, with bouts of depression, but with help and support he has completed two years at college and is looking forward to a third year.

Kate and Thelma feel that too often there is a 'check-list' approach to the problems young people have and, as Kate says, 'They don't always fit in boxes, do they?'

This is an important lesson for all those who provide services 'at the interface'. Although the young man Thelma cares for is now moving into independent living, she is aware that he will still have his ups and downs: 'We know we will be supporting him for the rest of his life.'

Thelma and Kate feel that foster carers have been able to speak with authority about independent living and have made a difference to how professionals think about services for looked-after children 'post-16'. 'After all,' Thelma says, 'you don't put your own child on the street at 16.'

## Advisory role on training

Kate and Thelma are acutely aware of the training needs of carers, especially around sexual abuse. Thelma, who fosters young males who have been sexually abused, had requested training on this subject on a number of occasions, with the result that the National Society for the Prevention of Cruelty to Children (NSPCC) did some training on young people who engage in sexually harmful behaviour. Thelma was asked to advise on the areas that she felt carers would need to have covered. She then wrote a list and the trainers made sure those areas were included.

## Advice on secondary trauma

Thelma feels that carers have a particularly important role in informing others about the experience of being a carer and the impact of some experiences that carers have.

'Secondary trauma' is a common term for trauma experienced at second hand, so to speak, through exposure to traumatic experiences as a professional. It is often experienced by those working with and caring for abused and traumatised children. However, there can be other traumas too, as Thelma knows only too well. Four years ago, one of the young men she was caring for hung himself. This highlighted for Thelma the issue of counselling and support for carers. She is determined to pursue counselling for carers who have experienced trauma, and feels this should be routinely available to them, just as it is for social workers. After taking up this issue with the Assistant Director, she has been assured that it will be taken forward.

Despite her continuing sadness, Thelma is able to think and talk about what she learned from this young person and how this understanding has helped other children she has cared for to survive. She says of the young man who died, 'We learned so much from him.'

## Therapy as consultation

In recent years, there has been a growing awareness of the therapeutic needs of young people who are 'looked after' and who have often experienced repeated broken attachments, as well as the trauma of abuse and neglect. Research evidence tells us that such children benefit most from therapeutic experiences that promote positive attachment experiences with their carers, whilst enabling them to grieve their past losses (Hughes 1998). Much of this work is undertaken with the child and carer together.

Thelma and Kate, like many other carers, have been regularly involved in such therapeutic experiences and have shared the often harrowing therapeutic journeys towards recovery with many of their children. Sometimes, the work is more consultative. Kate describes this as a process of shared understanding, with the therapist and carer working together. Like all of us, there have been times when she has found herself feeling defeated by a problem. She describes telling her therapist, 'I've come to a brick wall', and his response being, reassuringly, 'There's no problem with that Kate: we do that as well.' This therapist's respect for Kate's day-to-day work with children and his acknowledgement of her expertness helped her to go on.

Kate and Thelma try to use their experiences of therapeutic work with children, as well as their wealth of caring experiences that are, in themselves, therapeutic, to help other carers. Kate described how at a carers' meeting she had been chatting to Thelma about a child when a 'new' carer (who had been caring for about six months) sitting next to her began to talk of some of the fears she had. Kate was able to help this carer by suggesting, 'You don't need to be frightened. Don't look at the behaviour: look underneath it and over time the frightening behaviour will stop.'

It seems appropriate to end this chapter with a poem by Kate.

> A Child Lost
>
> Here is a child with nowhere to go,
> They'll stand and tremble from head to toe,
> There's an inner hurt deep down inside,
> It's filled with anger they just can't hide.
>
> They'll stand in silence without a word,
> Because their words are rarely heard,

There's no one there to ease the pain,
Their crying and weeping seem all in vain.

They'll punish themselves whenever they can,
And hold their feelings for a lifetime's span,
They would love to scream and let themselves go,
It would set them free and this they know.

But their feelings won't go without a fight,
They'll struggle and hold them with all their might.
To find a trust and feel they belong
And move in a world lighthearted as song
Would lighten the soul of this struggling child,
And make them secure and gentle and mild.

Kate Stokes, September 2001

## Further information

**Thelma Barlow** and **Kate Stokes** can be contacted through Pete Gray, Service Co-ordinator, SUSTAIN, Unit 2, Mill Bank Surgery, Mill Bank, Stafford ST16 2AG.

**The Jigsaw Group** can be contacted through Machita Denny on 07949691945 or at Trust Headquarters, St George's Hospital, Corporation Street, Stafford.

**Cannock Chase Young People's Group** can be contacted at Cannock Chase CAMHS, Crown House, Beecroft Road, Cannock, Staffs WS11 1JP.

For more information about the short films made by the young people and film-making workshops in general, contact info@digitalstories.info.

## References

Clarke C, Boateng P and Hodge M (2003) *Every Child Matters*. DFES Publications, London.
Green S (2004) *South Staffs Healthcare NHS Trust: Heart of the Trust Scheme Evaluation*. South Staffs Healthcare NHS Trust.
Hughes DA (1998) *Building the Bonds of Attachment*. Jason Aronson, Inc., Northvale.

# Chapter 13

# A new approach to consultation

*Angela Southall*

Consultation is perhaps best described as an explorative process that is shared by consultant and consultee. It seems to work best when the climate is one of mutual appreciation, each valuing what the other has to offer. Sinclair and Epps, in Chapter 9, make an important distinction of consultation *with* as opposed to *to* others. This suggests something about the consultation relationship being one between equal participants. However, the continuing culture of expertism often seems to militate against this by supporting the established professional hierarchy, something that is also inherent in the child and adolescent mental health service (CAMHS) tiered structure (*see* Chapter 6).

There are undoubtedly many contradictions, ambiguities and dilemmas around the idea of expertness. It is self-evident that consultation has to be useful, otherwise why bother to engage in such a process? The consultee (whether individual, group or organisation) will usually want to consult someone who can help them in a particular way. For example, residential staff at a children's unit are likely to want to consult with a practitioner who is experienced in working with looked-after children whilst the health visitor would probably value working with someone who has a grounding in child development, as well as attachment and family work. This suggests that we should not be shy about our areas of expertise. However, there is a difference between being able to draw upon some expert knowledge and adopting the stance of being an expert. Arguably, it is the ability to do the former without adopting the stance of the latter that makes us better consultants. Further, it seems clear that the skills needed to do this effectively do not seem to belong to any single profession. Nor do they reside within any particular 'domain' of expertise, as Evan George demonstrates in his chapter on solution-focused consultation (*see* Chapter 4).

## Consultation and containment

A recurrent theme of this book is that of containment. One of the most important characteristics of effective consultation, in fact, seems to be its containing function, that is, its function as a 'holding' exercise. The consultant tries to understand what the consultee is experiencing through the conversation, accepts these experiences and reflects them back to the consultee, in a way that helps him or her to make sense of them and to move forward from what often feels to be a 'stuck' position. The consultation must be therefore experienced as safe enough for both parties to be able 'to be, rather than to do' and to tolerate uncertainty. There is often value in making explicit the uncertainty and position of not knowing, especially on those occasions that 'the answer' is obviously and vigorously sought. Similarly, it is helpful to acknowledge the difficulty or complexity of the problem, holding this, rather than hurrying it to a conclusion.

These conditions are difficult to meet when there is pressure to act, as there often is. In these cases, the consultee is likely to feel impatient and pressured. The response will be, 'Just do it for me: I haven't got time to learn how to do it myself.' Such responses are inevitable in organisations that do not value consultation or see it merely as an 'add-on' to other services.

This brings us to a very important consideration. What happens when individual or organisational issues become highlighted through the consultation process? As a result of the conversation between consultant and consultee, issues may emerge that are matters for the individual to pursue through their own supervision. Examples include difficulties with specific types of case-work, working outside professional competencies or being overloaded with too much work. If such difficulties are identified, there must be an appropriate pathway for them to be taken up. It is essential that the consultant is able to assume the consultee to be a competent practitioner working within the limits of their role and with appropriate supervision and support systems (and vice versa, of course). It is also the case that organisational issues may become highlighted through the consultation process and this can prove difficult for the consultant if there are no agreed mechanisms for such discussions to take place. It could be argued that the organisation that changes only at the level of individual practice does not change at all.

## What consultation offers (and what it doesn't)

Consultation is not a cure-all. Neither is it the solution to the problems experienced by health, social care and education systems that are experiencing chronic problems of resource and capacity. These problems need careful analysis and brave solutions that challenge the self-perpetuation of systems and processes that are resistant to change and accommodate instead to the changing contexts around them. What consultation offers is an opportunity to do things differently, as well as more effectively, and to gain insights that contribute to what should be an ongoing process of change and development. It could be argued that consultation should be a thread running through all services in CAMHS – the wider CAMHS, that is, not just the community CAMHS teams – and, further, that it should be the strongest thread.

Through the varied chapters in this text, it is possible to draw a number of conclusions about consultation, which can be summarised as follows:

- Consultation is not a panacea.
- It helps people discover strengths and skills they didn't realise they had.
- It also helps draw out key areas for development, both in the individual and for the organisation.
- Consultation is essentially about containment; it is a containing relationship.
- Interagency consultation can lead to improved understanding and better working relationships between agencies – but this cannot be assumed as 'given'.
- It needs dedicated time.

- It uses a different set of skills to those used in clinical/case-work, which training is needed to develop. Not everyone can do it.
- When successful, consultation is a good use of time for all concerned.
- It does not necessarily lead to a reduction in workload, but may do so.

## Towards a new theory of consultation

The CAMHS tiered model is problematic in terms of its conceptualisation, not only in the way it mixes services and functions but also in the way it is interpreted. The model also helps perpetuate the idea that less skilled work is needed to deliver services at the lower tiers, such as 1 or 2, than at the higher ones (3 or 4). Although practitioners working at these levels know that this is not the case, they often have a difficult time persuading others who have limited experience of working in the community or with other agencies. This is sometimes especially true of those holding the purse strings. Such a view is unfortunate. Not only does the hierarchical interpretation lead to a degradation of consultation work, it contributes to the strong myth that anyone can do it. Hence, in many community CAMHS teams consultation work is given to the more junior or less experienced practitioners. As they do not have the requisite skills and experience to do the work, it either fails to develop or fails completely. Unfortunately, this is often understood in terms of a failure of consultation. As Banhatti and Dwivedi (Chapter 7) point out, consultation is not always 'to tier 1' and can be taking place in any setting. This suggests a non-linear, non-hierarchical process.

## The impact of consultation on services

A modern CAMHS requires qualified staff to be proficient in consultation skills, something that carries with it training implications. At the moment, few CAMHS practitioners undergo training in consultation; the training they do receive as part of their professional qualification does not equip them for this task. On the other hand *meta-professional* training, such as that exemplified by systemic and solution-focused approaches, offers new possibilities, using similar skills and techniques to help move from problem to solution, whatever the context. This suggests that professional training requirements need to change and adapt to new circumstances, training not just in 'doing' but also 'facilitating'.

The editor of this text has presided over developments in a community CAMHS team that has moved to – and maintained – a position of having no waiting list. This has not been the result of just one individual element but it is fair to say that consultation has featured very much in this, along with integration of solution-focused approaches into the model of working. All in all, it has been the creation of a different culture and much more of a commitment to the growth and development of work in (and by) the community.

Community psychology means not only taking services *out there*: it is a 'whole community' approach that sees services and partnerships as contributing to the growth of healthy communities. Such a philosophy views mental health as everyone's business and consultation a key element in supporting others to make it so. Arguably, consultation also challenges the 'treatment' model in mental health, as Michael Foulkes suggests in Chapter 6, replacing it with one of support and validation. It is something of an understatement to describe this as a mere mind-shift.

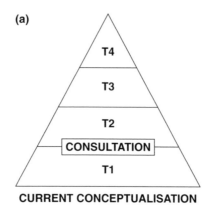

**(a)**

CURRENT CONCEPTUALISATION

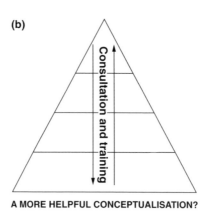

**(b)**

A MORE HELPFUL CONCEPTUALISATION?

**Figure 13.1** (a) Although consultation does not happen exclusively at the T1–T2 inter-face, this is where the major focus is deemed to be; (b) This figure shows consultation happening 'up and down' the tiers (e.g. social workers consulting with specialist CAMHS practitioners on such things as child protection and life-story work, educational psychologists consulting with workers up and down the tiers on helping with attention motivation and concentration difficulties, and so on).

## Conclusion

The 'hands on' experiences described in this text suggest that consultation has a considerable potential contribution to services, over and above facilitating practice, promoting mutual understanding and highlighting training needs. It can give rise to genuinely needs-led service developments and be a driver for change. There is a strong argument for placing consultation at the centre of services – not at the periphery. It is hoped that this book will help that process and will serve as a contribution towards developing a new model of consultation that is process-orientated and facilitative of development and change – whether applied to professionals, organisations and systems or service users. Amidst services that seem to be more and more target driven, we are all prey to the same forces of business and busy-ness. To consult effectively, as we have seen, requires a set of skills that sometimes seem to be pulling us in the opposite direction. It also requires us to think, rather than to react. And the difference is in the thinking. If, whilst reading this, you have found yourself enjoying the idea but wondering how you are going to really find the time for it (or to do more of it, perhaps, or take it to a different level), maybe now is a good time to stop and think.

# Index

Page numbers in *italics* refer to case studies or tables